A Basic History of Nursing

Second edition

JM Mellish
DN BA MCur (Ed) MCur (Admin) DCur RGN RM
Emeritus Professor of Nursing Science
University of Port Elizabeth

Butterworths
Durban

Butterworths
Professional Publishers (Pty) Ltd
Reg No 87/03997/07

First edition 1984

ISBN 0 409 10011 0

Durban
8 Walter Place, Waterval Park
Mayville 4091

Johannesburg
108 Elizabeth Avenue
Benmore 2010

Pretoria
301 Telkor Building, 270 Main Street
Waterkloof 0181

Cape Town
3 Gardens Business Village, Hope Street
Cape Town 8001

Artefacts used for the cover photography kindly supplied by the
Addington Archives and Museum Society, Durban.

Typeset by Adcolour Pinetown
Printed and bound by Interpak (Natal) Pietermaritzburg
The imprint Butterworths is used under licence

Preface

This text has been prepared in response to numerous requests for a straight-forward basic history of nursing which is readily available, includes an overview of the history of nursing in South Africa, and is suitable for diploma students and others who want an introduction to the subject.

The author's indebtedness to numerous researchers of and writers on the subject over many years, those who gave direction to her own studies, and in particular to Professor Charlotte Searle for her tremendous contribution to knowledge of the history of nursing in South Africa, is acknowledged with gratitude.

This second edition includes some new material, has been updated and aims at making modern nurses realise that nursing is done by people, caring for other people, and that people have not changed to such a great extent throughout the ages.

JM Mellish

Contents

Preface

1

PRIMITIVE TIMES

1.1 Introduction

History is about people; without people history is nothing. The people in history are physically much the same as we are today. People are conceived and born in much the same way as the original human inhabitants of the earth, with the exception that modern science and technology may be used not only to remove the baby surgically from the womb by 'Caesarean section', but also to ensure the survival of the mother.

The name *Caesarean section* is actually derived from the tradition that Julius Caesar or one of his ancestors was born by such an operation from the incised womb of his mother. There is no actual historical proof of this, but the legend lives on.

From the beginning of time the human race has been characterised by its *physical* body. Man has a skeleton forming a framework covered by tissues, muscles that enable various parts to move, a heart that pumps blood through arteries and veins to all parts of the body. He has a respiratory system which allows him to breathe, digestive organs that process food taken in by the mouth and make it available for use by the tissues, and excrete the waste products.

The actual food that was consumed in early times may have been different in many ways, but if one thinks about it, so is the food taken by different people in different parts of the world today. Nonetheless the digestive process is the same as it always has been, and the basic food requirements remain the same.

Man, the human body, has a urinary system that rids the body of waste products; he has a brain and nerves that travel to all parts of the body. The brain in the human being is larger than that of any other animal and is the source of man's intellect. Male and female reproductive systems differ to allow for the reproduction of the species; this has always been so. There is also an endocrine system with its many specialised functions.

Man has always had the basic anatomical structure and physiological processes which enable him to function as man, a member of the human race.

When reading the following chapters or any other historical text, one should always try to remember that we are reading about people who actually lived and died on this planet.

Since the beginning of time men, women and children have been susceptible to illnesses. Growing scientific knowledge has, however, altered the management of diseases and the causes of many have only become known in recent times, even though they have always existed. If cut, men bleed, bones have always been susceptible to being broken from various causes, and the basic healing pattern remains the same.

Men as we well know are different in many ways. No two people are ever exactly alike, not even identical twins. They have different skin pigmentation and hair of different texture and colour. Their build may vary from tall to very short or even dwarf-like (dwarfs are shown in many ancient pictures, they are no new phenomenon), stocky or slim, thin or fat, young and old.

Man has always been dependent on shelter from the elements and has made use of his brain and nimble fingers to develop different forms of shelter. This was based on the climate, available materials and the level of sophistication of the times. Clay huts, straw huts, caves, hide tents and wooden buildings all preceded the more elaborate stone and brick buildings. Some of these ancient buildings were very well built and are still evident today. Through the course of time the basic human being has remained.

History is not to be equated to a dull memorisation of dates. Although dates are important with regard to *when* events occurred in the past (events in different parts of the world at a certain time should be seen in relation to each other), but learning dates without considering the actual *people* who were alive at the time, and *how* they were *affected* by what happened around them, has no meaning. When we study history, we must try to see the life of the people living in the past in relation to the events in other centuries and try to gain perspective of our own time through what has happened in the past.

Some chronological order will be maintained in the text, but the fascinating subject of the history of nursing can be viewed from many points of view. It is more than an accumulation of facts, set out in chronological order. The student of history must become aware of trends in events which have shaped the practice of nursing and on which its philosophy has been based. She should become conscious of herself as being part of the history of nursing. An awareness of what has gone before, what has been achieved by those who have preceded the nurse of today, and a pride in her profession, built on the past but pointing to the future, should be evoked.

At the same time it must be pointed out that interpretations of events will differ according to the values and norms of one's own culture and times and the changing values which are part of a dynamic society and a dynamic profession.

In this life nothing is in limbo, everything and everyone is related in some way to the past, which also has an influence on the future. This is as true of the human race as it is of the history of a particular area, country, continent, a specific race or a specific profession.

This work will attempt to give a broad overview of the history of a specific profession – *nursing* – in the hope that it will stimulate further reading, where readers may discover the fascinating, rich pattern of nursing history for themselves and build on this through their own interpretations and understanding.

The source of material on which history is based is varied and widespread. The past has gone and the far distant past has been gone for a very long time indeed. One cannot recover what has been lost. Written records date only from the time when language had evolved and man developed the means of writing about events. Art forms, rock paintings, the uncovering of artefacts from bygone ages by archaeologists, and the work done by sociologists and anthropologists among primitive tribes that have been 'discovered' in recent times have all contributed to creating an image of what life must have been like in primitive times.

History is, by definition, 'an account of an event; a systematic account of the origin and progress of the world, a nation, an institution, a science, etc; a knowledge of past events' (41:594).

If there was no writing to record events, the only way in which events of the past could be made known to future generations was by word of mouth. This, of course, excludes the paintings of occurrences or their depiction in sculpture.

If the reader pauses to think of descriptions of events at which she was actually present, she will soon acknowledge that oral representations of the past are often not as she remembers them, and that certain points are highlighted while others are left out, according to the personal impressions of the person recounting the event. Legends are still born amongst us every day, and they grow and alter with the telling. A good storyteller often unconsciously embellishes his story to make it more interesting or more dramatic. Thus oral 'history' cannot be relied on as always being accurate. Far from it. On careful consideration one will realise that written records can to some extent suffer from the same distortion too. What appears important to one recorder may seem completely insignificant to another. Thus such evidence as exists has to be sifted and compared before any conclusions can be drawn.

When sifting through ancient writings one also has to bear in mind that they were written in ancient languages, and are therefore difficult to translate into the languages of today. For instance, scholars are constantly uncovering inaccuracies in the translation of the Bible. Everyday usage has also changed the original meaning of words in our own language, creating misconceptions.

If the reader keeps these observations in mind, then the study of the history of nursing (or any other history) becomes a constant, exciting voyage of discovery. This voyage will be coloured not only by the writer, whose own background, values and norms must influence the writing, but also by the background, values and norms of the student and the cultural patterns of the society in which she has been nurtured.

History is not a dry-as-dust past, something which is dead. Alternatively, it is something which was alive and vital to those living in the times described; as alive and vital as events of today are to those living in today's world, which is in any case tomorrow's yesterday.

In an occasional paper in the *Nursing Times* (34), Marion Ferguson states that knowledge of a history of their craft is central to nurses' understanding and to their practice within the health care structure. She maintains that the implications of events are crucial for the practice of nursing and not the events *per se*.

In preparing this text the writer has consulted many sources and direct acknowledgement will be made where appropriate. However, these sources are of necessity secondary sources. The point of view which will be followed will be that health and disease have been present in man from time immemorial, and that a means of dealing with deviations from health existed before the dawn of the scientific era.

Nursing has been interwoven with other forms of health care and has indeed often preceded them and has varied in its application and meaning throughout the ages. Some chronological form will be maintained to give order to the whole text, but nursing history will be looked at as a phenomenon interlinked with being human and not just as a record of the past. It arose to meet the special needs of human beings throughout the ages. These needs have varied greatly, just as they do today, according to many circumstances, climatic conditions and other factors, but *people* meeting the needs of other *people* have always been involved.

1.2 Pre-history

The history of nursing before the time of written records can only be based on speculation on what has been gathered from the research into 'newly discovered' primitive tribes, and from artefacts, rock paintings and the like. Pots and tools, houses and tombs, weapons and ornaments have been dug up and uncovered by archaeological research. Prehistoric times are characterised by the non-existence of writing, all over the world. As time passed, non-literate peoples, that is, peoples who had no written language, existed side by side with those who had already developed some form of writing. This does not mean that all members of the group could write. Such anomalies continue even today and illiteracy is still very prevalent, especially in the Third World. Furthermore, sophisticated treatment of sick people exists alongside folk medicine and magic practices even in the late 20th century.

Archaeologists have been able to demonstrate the superimposition of the remains of one culture on another in the same area. History itself is said to begin when writing began. From present evidence, this appears to be about 3 000 years before the Christian Era (BCE) in Mesopotamia.

Evidence has been found that man may have existed on this planet over a million years ago. *Homo sapiens* first appeared between 30 000 and 40 000 years ago (24:21). The same source states that the first toolmaking humans of whom there is a clear picture lived about 4 000 000 years ago. These remains were found near Peking, now Beijing. They were about 1,5 m tall and had learnt to make fire, were hunters, and had started making tools. By 25000 BCE *Homo sapiens* was also making objects which were used to adorn his body. Small figurines of women have also been found over a wide area. Gradually humans emerged from being cage dwellers, made skin tents and clothed themselves in skins from animals which they hunted for food.

In this period of time the human being was living, giving birth and dying. Compared with the many huge animals, the mammoths, and ferocious beasts which he hunted for food, he was a frail creature. His body was slight and unprotected, and he had to devise his own defence against the elements. His greatest assets were his nimble fingers and his large brain, which enabled him to outwit the larger animals with whom he shared the planet.

It was during this time that the *primitive mother*, as we think of her today, must have existed. A mother gave birth to her child, fed and nurtured him as he grew up, protected him from danger until he could fend for himself, and looked after him when he suffered injury or illness. A woman would have lived with her man and raised a family. Because the man had to hunt for food, it is probable that he would have been injured at some time, and the woman would have naturally been the one to do her best to look after him and other members of the family unit. He could have, for example, been burned by fire and injured by warring tribes or falls, natural disasters and other mishaps.

Cave paintings have been found depicting women giving birth, and it appears likely that these women helped each other when the need arose.

As man developed through the ages, so did his skills and his civilisation. Piggot's definition (24:11) of civilisation follows.

> [Civilisation is] a society which has worked out a solution to the problems of living in a relatively large community, at a level of technological development above that of the hunting band, the family farmstead, the rustic self-sufficient village or the pastoral tribe. Civilisation is something artificial and man-made, the result of making tools of increasing complexity in response to the enlarging concepts of community life evolving in men's minds.

This definition may be somewhat lengthy, but enables the reader to see clearly how nursing could have developed in such a context, from primitive mother to the nurse in the space age.

Between 8000 and 7000 BCE man began to build huts and houses, domesticated the dog and the goat, and discovered the art of reaping and storing grain. Agriculture possibly developed about 7000 to 6500 BCE and villages and towns started to develop. This means that life became more settled and some form of social organisation emerged, with definite tribal leaders. The dead were disposed of, often being buried under the dwelling place. Many ancient graves have been found in different parts of the world.

Baly (1:3) says that 'nursing must have developed as a response to changing social needs . . . which are continuous in the history of man'.

As communities grew, so the problems of community health must have followed. The fact that some answers must have been found to health hazards which existed at the time, is proved by the survival of the human race. Man required shelter from the elements. First he found shelter in caves, then he developed skills which enabled him to make hide tents, huts and houses. Clothes were made to protect himself. He developed tools for hunting and for his own use.

The growth of communities meant that water sources would have to be protected. Although he knew nothing of micro-organisms, he must have realised that disease followed the use of water from certain sources. Sanitation would have become a growing problem with which he had to contend. Food was hunted and gathered, and later deliberately grown.

The mother breastfed her baby. She also prepared food for her family and must have been aware of those substances which caused health problems such as vomiting or diarrhoea, that is, foods that 'did not agree with people' to use modern lay terminology. It seems to have been customary for the so-called 'wise women' of the tribe to collect the available natural substances such as plants, seeds, nuts, roots and the bark of trees for healing purposes. Some would be applied locally, while concoctions of extracts from others were probably prepared as oral medications. Knowledge of those that seemed to be of benefit must have been handed down from one generation to another. This we have experienced in the tribal medications of the indigenous people of our own country. We know, from contact with primitive peoples and developing communities, that many empirical remedies were used to treat pain, injury and illness.

The discovery of a Stone Age skull in Peru in 1860 by an American anthropologist, E Squier, was sent to Dr Paul Broca, an authority in physical anthropology (18:24). Broca confirmed that the trepanning which was carefully done, had occurred while the person was still alive. He also stated that the bone showed signs of infection, which meant that the person had lived for some two weeks after the operation at least. Many other skulls with similar patterning of trepanning have been found in numerous parts of the world. A large number showed the growth of healthy new bone, which seems to indicate that the operations which were carried out, not only on head injury cases (hunting/fighting accidents), but also on women and children, were successful.

Trepanning was still being carried out in the Pacific Islands well into the 20th century. The belief was held that fits, chronic headaches and depression were caused by evil spirits and that these 'bad' spirits could be released and replaced with 'good' spirits by making a hole in the skull. Imagine all the headaches and depression of modern times being treated in the same way! This Stone Age culture of the Pacific Islands gives us a clue as to what the inhabitants of the Stone Age must have believed.

Chipped or smoothed stone blades were used for these operations, such instruments having been found in the unearthing of Stone Age remains.

The rate of survival is gauged by the numbers of trepanned skulls which have been found, in which healing had taken place. No anaesthetics were used, although in Peru coca leaves (from which cocaine is derived) were chewed to alleviate pain. Some pain-killing medicines must have also been made from herbs and plants. Infection must have been less rife than it is today, or a very high resistance to infection had been built up in those who survived the primitive 'surgery' of the time. Operations without anaesthetics must have taken a long time to perform with a fully conscious or at least only semi-conscious patient, and meant that the person on whom the operation was being performed, (and who survived the operation), must have had an extremely high pain threshold.

Even to survive infancy meant that the individual was very tough physically at least (the survival of the fittest). One supposes that the umbilical cord was cut by a stone or a reed. No knowledge of sterilisation existed, although there must have been infective agents as seen from the bone that showed signs of infection after trepanning. The 20th century nurse may have difficulties to imagine all of this with the modern emphasis on asepsis, antisepsis and antibiotics and other means of treating infection if it does occur.

The Stone Age was followed by the Bronze Age with improvements in the types of instruments which were fashioned. Again, the development of these implements for surgery did not occur simultaneously or at the same rate in different parts of the world where there was no communication or sharing of such 'discoveries'. Thus, a Bronze Age culture would have evolved in one part of the world long before people in other areas had found the way to make instruments of metal.

Margotta (22:13) says that 'palaeontologists have revealed signs of pathological conditions in very ancient remains; injuries and diseases have always been hazards of living beings and man is as vulnerable as any other'.

Primitive mother would have had to deal with many ills and her influence and role in nurturing the young and caring for those who were struck by injury and disease would have spread from the family to the extended family, the clan and the tribe. This form of nursing takes place even today. It is a simple, practical form of caring for one's own and one's neighbours.

1.3 Beliefs regarding health and disease

According to Margotta (22:14), fossil remains 'show evidence of diseases such as arthritis and tuberculosis as well as bone deformities caused by injury'.

The relationship of injury to suffering must have been obvious, but how to explain suffering caused by disease which seemed to come from nowhere and was a threat to health and life must have presented problems. It is difficult for the sophisticated student who has completed 12 years of schooling to imagine such a situation, to envisage health care without hospitals, clinics, doctors, a huge armentarium of medications, X-rays, tests, and a wealth of written knowledge concerning disease, its causation and treatment. If she can just briefly try to imagine what life would have been like without all the trappings of late 20th-century health care, it will be easier to understand the seemingly weird and wonderful beliefs and practices that primitive man developed.

Man needed an explanation for many strange phenomena, for sudden inexplicable storms and for natural disasters as well as for incomprehensible illnesses. He thus came to believe in demon possession, evil spirits, and the need to propitiate gods or some other form of supernatural being, to explain the evils in one form or another which was visited on him, or members of his family, tribe or nation.

Alongside the empirical remedies developed by the wise women of the tribe by trial and error, and the *animistic* theory that inanimate objects and natural phenomena have living souls which can exert evil as well as good influences on human beings, a belief in the power of magic practices to counteract evil influences, developed.

The role of *shaman, medicine man* or *witchdoctor* emerged. This person was a sorcerer, a member of a class apart, who was thought to be possessed of supernatural powers. He could act for good as well as ill and was thought to be capable of weaving spells which could heal people. It was believed, he could also cast evil spells on people to make them ill. Consequently the lifting of evil spells was part of his stock-in-trade too. Many of the results must have been a combination of medications which had some efficacy, primitive surgery, and the psychosomatic effects of the rituals and 'treatments' performed by the medicine man.

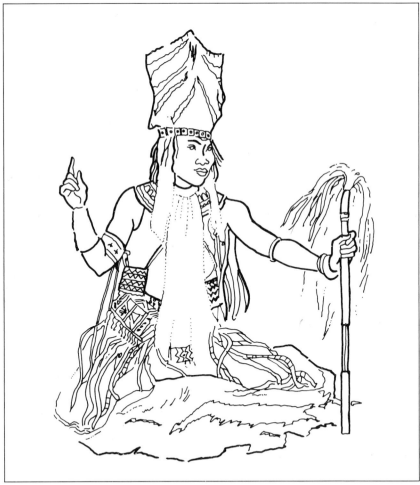

A traditional witchdoctor

Animal masks were worn to frighten away evil spirits, trephining of skulls was undertaken to let out these malicious spirits, or simply to relieve headache or epilepsy which was probably thought to have been caused by demon possession. The oldest instruments which have been found are sharpened stones which were apparently used to incise abscesses, to let blood and to trephine.

Mandrake was used as a soporific (it contains hyoscine) and according to Margotta (22:18) antidotes to snakebite go back to the 'dim and distant past'. Quinine obtained from the bark of the chinchona tree was used by primitives in Peru and the muscle relaxant curare was used by the native inhabitants of South America as an arrow poison.

Some of the practices, such as punching or kicking the patient, plunging him alternately into hot and cold water to scare evil spirits, or attempting to scare the baby from the body of a pregnant woman, would today be considered barbaric; yet some of these practices persist in remote areas even in the late 20th century.

Other methods employed in 'medical' practice were the wearing of charms to ward off evil spirits, and attempts to transfer these malicious beings or disease conditions to inanimate objects or animals. Belief in the efficacy of charms has not disappeared from so-called 'civilised' beings. 'Lucky' talismans are still worn, people still believe that the number 13 is unlucky, and many avoid walking under a ladder for the same reason. Superstitious beliefs are certainly not things of the past.

In the RSA 'witchdoctors' and the effects of their ministrations are still very evident. Distortion of ears for the insertion of adornments and the scarification caused by tribal markings can still be seen in the streets of our cities. The reality of such 'magic' practices is not difficult to grasp.

In an article in *Curationis* (40) van Rensburg says the following.

> [A] long established system of traditional medicine among blacks in South Africa exists alongside Westernised health services . . . evidence exists that it is still widely used and that the continued use of the traditional healers, often together with Western medicine, is rooted in traditionally held concepts of health and disease. Illness and death are usually attributed to mystical causes which must be identified and removed by the witch-doctor . . . It is not envisaged that the witch-doctor will cease to play a role in the foreseeable future.

The traditional healer still plays an important part in Southern Africa, evidence of their 'charms' being found on patients accepting Western medicine in hospitals. Many countries in Africa accept the status and role of the traditional healers. Karlsson and Motloantoa (33:26-29) state that traditional beliefs are important in that they explain not only *how* but also *why* an event occurs to the person. It is commonly believed that sorcerers can make the environment dangerous in various ways, for example, by scattering various 'harmful' substances in the path so that a specific person becomes ill after he has stepped on them.

These traditional healers have developed medicines which they use, derived mostly from herbs, barks and roots, which are usually collected fresh, while only a few of these medicines derive from animal sources. Illness is often perceived as being caused by some evil which has to be physically expelled from the patient's body, hence the extensive use of emetics, enemas and purgatives, which are used to 'cleanse' the body (33:28) before 'curative' medicines can be administered.

This is evidence of a primitive cultural pattern enduring into the late 20th century.

1.4 Recorded history – Early civilisations

Again the role of the nurse is largely a matter of conjecture, but recorded history has brought with it some knowledge of medical practices and it can safely be assumed that first-level nursing (the non-scientific mother role and the care given by members of the family, neighbours or friends) was practised. A brief look will be taken at some of the early civilisations, their general characteristics and health practices in an attempt to follow the evolution of the nurse to the present.

Much evidence has been gathered by researchers and synthesised by them from *hieroglyphic* inscriptions (a type of writing where figures or objects represented words, as found in ancient Egypt), *cuneiform* writings (wedge-shaped writings found in ancient Persia and Assyria), *papyri* (an ancient writing material prepared from the stems of an aquatic reed) and from old documents giving actual case histories, from paintings, sculpture and other artefacts.

When studying this section, the student must remember that more advanced civilisations existed alongside primitive peoples. All did not develop at the same rate, nor did all evolve in the same way, so that fairly advanced health care was practised in some civilisations, whereas it was completely lacking in others.

One must remember that communication was limited and travel was slow and difficult, besides being dangerous. On foot, mounted on horse or donkey or camel, if that was the animal used in that part of the world, movement from place to place was a lengthy, time-consuming process. Travelling by lake or sea was in rowing boats or boats which used primitive sails. There were no roads, and it took many years before the wheel was invented. Pulling sled-like carts preceded this development. Such sled-like carts are still used as a mode of transport in remote parts of our country, even in this day and age.

Men had little idea of their near neighbours and it took brave adventurers to set sail from their home territory. All this is difficult to relate to in a time where the telephone, telegraphs, fax machine, air travel and satellite transmission of images put us in touch with the rest of the world within hours, if not seconds, and we are able to see televised images of events in different parts of the world, or even from outer space as they are taking place, or immediately afterwards. The world may seem small to us, but its vastness is tremendous and must have been quite daunting to those who set sail for unknown climes.

Air, water and sea travel and transport are so extensively used in modern times, that we may take them for granted. There are of course still air, lake and sea disasters, but in relation to the number of hours travelled by millions of people and the amount of freight carried around the world, the dangers on such modes of transport in proportion to the cargo carried in ancient times in fragile boats, with no radar or radio communication, is infinitesimal.

At the same time it must be remembered that the number of people inhabiting the world has also increased dramatically, in addition to all the prevalent health problems that this has brought with it.

Literacy in its various forms also developed at different rates among different people at different times. One only has to compare Japanese brush writing with the typeface in this text to understand this point.

1.4.1 The Sumerians

According to Mallowan (24:67) 'the first light of civilisation dawned in the fertile valleys of the Tigris and Euphrates in the centuries around 4000 BCE'. Others state that this was a full 1 000 years earlier.

These rivers flow through the present-day Turkey, Syria and Iraq, join near Basra and enter the Persian Gulf as the Shatt-al-Arab River which flows along the Iraqi-Iranian border.

The oldest picture writing (dated about 3500 BCE) was found at Kish, situated 88 km south of modern Baghdad in Sumeria (now part of Iraq). Sumeria was the term the ancient Semites or Akkadians of Mesopotamia used to denote the area of the lower valley of the Tigris and Euphrates south of Babylon (32:5151). The Sumerians appear to have entered Mesopotamia and conquered the land from the Semites in the fourth century BCE. About 25 000 clay tablets, 95 per cent of which are economic in nature, have been discovered and give evidence of an advanced civilisation.

The Sumerians built their houses of sun-dried brick. (18:39). They believed that different gods ruled different cities and they built temples on the top of stepped pyramids made of brick for the worship and propitiation of these gods.

The first writings of this period were in the form of stylised drawings (pictographs) which were initially scratched on stone. A great deal of clay was available and it was found that 'writing' on clay with a reed was easier and the clay tablet could thereafter be dried in the sun. The pictures gradually developed into a form of writing.

Agriculture developed during this time and food supplies became more readily available. The diet was probably healthy and varied, consisting of wheat and barley which was ground into a coarse flour and baked into flat cakes in clay ovens. From their immediate environment the Sumerians gathered fruits and nuts where these were available. Meat was supplied from hunting and later from domesticated animals. Fishing was also practised.

Ur of the Chaldees as it is called in the book of Genesis in the Bible was a Sumerian city, situated on a bank of the river Euphrates. This city is best remembered as the birthplace of Abraham and was a flourishing city in 2 000 BCE. Tombs containing many bodies with beautiful artefacts were found dating from about 2 500 BCE.

Although the oldest known medical practices are those of the Sumerian civilisation, they were probably preceded by others, about which we have no written historical records. It is from this time that the link between religion and medicine developed. Temples were built as priesthood evolved. Perhaps the priest-physician concept had its origins in these days. Writing certainly first made its appearance in temples.

There was continuous war between cities, as well as political struggles for power. Community enterprises such as the digging of canals and the building of reservoirs (which had to be cleaned and kept in repair) were firmly established. Sumerian medicine was based on the study of astronomy, due to the belief that man's destiny was linked with the stars from the time of his birth.

According to Margotta (22:20,21) many clay tablets . . found in Sumeria were 'those used by priests for writing medical treatises in cuneiform script. Blood was thought to be the origin of every vital function. The liver was thought to be the collecting centre for blood, so that it was regarded as the *seat of life*.'

It was this belief that gave rise to the practice of trying to foretell portents for the future by the examination of the lobes of animal livers. Human sacrifice was practised – those serving royalty accompanied their superiors to the next world.

The Sumerian civilisation lasted until about 2000 BCE before being assimilated by the Assyrians and Babylonians who conquered Mesopotamia.

1.4.2 The Babylonians

The Assyrians and Babylonians conquered Mesopotamia and absorbed the Sumerian civilisation. The civilisations which they established lasted from about 2500 BCE until 560 BCE. Babylon, the centre of the Babylonian empire, was actually founded in about 3000 BCE and became the capital of Babylonia when this emerged as a distinct civilisation. Babylon was situated on the river Euphrates, about 80 km south of Baghdad in Iraq. The golden age of the Babylonian empire apparently lasted from 1750 until 562 BCE. Hammurabi, who was in power from 1728 to 1686 BCE, was a distinguished ruler who left behind him a code of laws (32:2586). Several copies of this code still exist on clay tablets and also on a black stone tablet about 2,5 metres high on which the laws are inscribed in cuneiform (wedge-shaped) characters.

This code represented a type of penal law, stating rewards and punishments, from which evidence on medical practices could be gleaned. For instance, if a surgeon performed a successful operation he was given his fee but if the patient died, one of the surgeon's hands was chopped off! Operations for officials of high rank also had to be performed at a cheaper rate than for ordinary citizens.

Since surgeons were laymen they were governed by the civil code, whereas physicians were priests, answerable to the gods. This code of laws, which laid down fees and penalties for surgeons, was probably the first in history (22:23) to define the concept of a surgeon's civil and criminal liability, incompetence or negligence being subject to punishment. It must have been a daunting prospect which faced surgeons who failed, and would have restricted their activities to a great extent.

Interesting to note is that Abraham, who was a descendant of Noah, lived at the same time as Hammurabi. The biblical flood appears to have been described in 12 tablets found under the king's temple at Nineveh (capital of the Assyrian empire). The biblical flood may be ascribed to a sudden and extraordinary flood in the Euphrates valley accompanied by heavy rain. Excavations in Mesopotamia show actual evidence of many severe floods which had occurred at different times.

It was still the belief that disease was caused by demons and the priest-physicians were said to interpret the actions of the demons and to call on the gods to alleviate the sufferings of the afflicted. It was also believed that some evil spirits were of human origin.

The oldest god with a medical connection was the moon god Sin, who supposedly made herbs grow and was believed to be able to destroy evil spirits. Later a god named Marduk was credited with the power to cure illness and inspire magical spells. Still later, different gods 'started specialisation' so that each was thought capable of curing some specific illness (22:21).

Known diseases in Babylonian times were tuberculosis, apoplexy, plague, rheumatism and venereal disease, while some tablets also have descriptions of diseases of the eyes, ears, skin and heart. Toothache was thought to be caused by the gnawing of a worm. Indeed, this was a common belief in Europe until the late 17th century (22:22).

It is also likely that the part played by insects in the spread of infectious diseases was recognised even at this early stage, while a wide range of drugs, including some minerals, was apparently prescribed. Primitive public health measures of the time, such as large stone drains, have also been excavated in Babylonia (22:24).

No mention is made of nurses as a separate category, but temple attendants probably assisted physicians by caring for their 'patients'. Since slavery was commonly practiced, it is also quite possible that slaves were used to care for the sick. Again this is pure conjecture, but a legitimate supposition.

Babylon was destroyed by the Assyrians under Sennacherib, before being rebuilt and becoming famous again during the rule of Nebuchadnezzar (605-581 BCE). It was a city of great luxury, and the famous 'hanging gardens' were built during this period.

The Greek historian Herodotus, who lived from about 484 to 424 BCE, visited Asia Minor including Mesopotamia (among other countries) and described the city of Babylon as follows.

> Next in ingenuity . . . is their treatment of disease. They have no doctors, but bring their invalids out into the street, where anyone who comes along offers the sufferer advice on his complaint, either from personal experience or observation of a similar complaint in others.

He also states that no one was allowed to pass a sick person in silence but had to at least enquire about the nature of his illness. The passer-by would then suggest remedies which he had known to be effective in other cases. A true *community* participation! He also writes that they buried their dead in honey, and describes hygienic practices (16:94).

1.4.3 The Assyrians

Assyria, an ancient state of Mesopotamia, was situated largely in the valley of the upper Tigris River and the mountains bordering it, in what is today known as Iraq. The civilisation existed roughly from 1750 to 650 BCE with some breaks. According to Lissner (21:43) the Assyrians, a Semitic tribe, were a tough, hardy race who fought against the Babylonians for hundreds of years. They were ferocious, fearless conquerors whose constant wars must have resulted in many injuries. A description of the life and times of Sennacherib (705-681 BCE), a brutal leader, is described on tablets found in the Royal Library of Nineveh by Layard and Rassan (32:365). These tablets go back to Sumerian times and cover the whole range of Assyrian learning and not only that of Sennacherib's lifetime. According to the same source they included 'medical treatises, with prescriptions, diagnosis, prognosis and treatment of all manner of disease'. Art forms such as reliefs on massive slabs depicted religious scenes with eagle-masked priests and 'sacred trees', from which the king was supposed to draw life for his people. The religion was pantheistic, and the many gods each had their own specific symbols, shrines and temples.

1.4.4 The ancient Egyptians

Cyril Aldred (24:99) states that the seeds of Egyptian civilisation were sown in the Nile Valley 6 000 years ago. There was a narrow strip of fertile land and it was here that the earliest traces of life dated about 5000 BCE have been found. The Egyptian peoples, co-existing as they did with other groups who were developing simultaneously in other areas, were cut off from outside influence by the sea and by deserts. The land was thus isolated from invaders and could develop in relative peace. Archaeological evidence dated about 3800 BCE, suggests that women and children tilled the fields with some masculine assistance, while the men still practised a certain amount of hunting. Apparently the chief of the tribe was also a medicine man and rain-maker. Fertility rites were practised.

During the 400 years following 3200 BCE, a distinct civilisation under one king (the *Pharaoh*) emerged. He was regarded as a 'god-king'. Arts and sciences flourished, writing became advanced and a flexible paper made of the papyrus reed was used. This made record-keeping possible, instructions could be sent throughout the land and history could be written down and thus preserved for future generations.

Casson (4:12) says 'medical science may have been said to have begun in Egypt. Though their knowledge was at times tainted with magic, the Egyptian doctors and surgeons of antiquity achieved international renown.' Egyptian people of ancient times also seem to have been 'sociable and lighthearted', and among the most industrious of ancient peoples' (4:14). They enjoyed life and believed in a life after death. The Nile was the nucleus of Egyptian economy.

Provided that it flooded each year, food was plentiful. It was the source of water for the cultivation of grain, raising of cattle, goats and pigs and for the geese, ducks and cranes which could be hunted for food. Food and other goods could be distributed along its course and fish abounded. Therefore, the people of Egypt must have at least had adequate nutrition. Egypt eventually expanded by conquest of other lands and the empire, which stretched right up to the Euphrates in the north, was consolidated in about 1450 BCE.

Imhotep, who lived around about 2800 BCE, was a famous architect who was also credited with being a writer and a physician. He created the *Step Pyramid*, as the tomb for Djosser at Sakkaia. This was the forerunner of the true pyramids.

From the decorations in the pyramids, the writings on papyri and the deciphering of hieroglyphics, it has been possible to piece together the medical history of the time. By about the seventh century BCE, that is long after his death, Imhotep was worshipped as the God of Medicine, and was later linked with Asklepios by the Greeks.

Herodotus visited Egypt and described the medicine of the Nile Valley, recording that although there were many physicians each specialised in one disease only.

The most famous of the so-called 'medical papyri' are those found by Ebers (the Ebers Medical Papyri), dated at about 1553-1550 BCE. They are a collection of old texts which originate from the old empire. According to Casson (4:148) these papyri seem to have been a kind of teaching manual for general practitioners, including even a section on speculative medical philosophy and one on pharmacy. There is also a surgical section as well as one on the heart and its vessels. The papyrus found by Smith known as the Edwin Smith Papyrus, is also a 'textbook' of the time and describes among others the treatment of fractures by splints, reduction of dislocations and the dressing of wounds, their clamping, suturing or joining with some form of adhesive paste. The examination of mummified bodies has shown that many healed without complications.

Casson (4:148) describes how Egyptian doctors *questioned* patients, *inspected* them and then carried out *functional tests*. They then *diagnosed* and decided either 'to treat' or 'to contend', that is, to 'struggle with' or 'not to treat'. It was also noted that lesions on the head were associated with paralysis on the opposite side of the body. Today we take such knowledge for granted, but if we place it in the context of 4 000 years ago, then the discernment of the 'doctors' of those long gone times was quite remarkable. Another famous medical papyrus was unearthed by Brughsch.

The Egyptians knew that the heart was the centre of circulation, but believed that circulation was dependent on respiration. They recognised diseases of the heart, abdomen, eyes and bladder and advised surgery for certain tumours. They also advocated cauterisation after surgery to prevent bleeding. The physicians appear to have visited their patients, taking the pulse and listening to the chest sounds by putting their ears over shoulder blades and the thorax.

There appear to have been priest-physicians who ministered to the living in the 'house of life', and another class of worker who prepared bodies for mummification. These worked in the 'house of death'. This separation of duties resulted in the priest-physicians not knowing as much of human anatomy as might have been supposed. They relied more on animal studies which of course did not give them completely accurate information, since animal anatomy often differs from that of humans (22:25-28). However, the study of mummified remains from ancient tombs gives present-day researchers a good insight into 'ancient' diseases. For instance, microscopic tissue study has given clear indications not only of bone lesions, but also of diseases such as arteriosclerosis. Many bodies have been found from ancient times which were not embalmed, but were preserved in the sand in the very dry climate of Egypt (8:20).

The ancient Egyptians seem to have suffered a great deal from dental problems, among which was the wearing down of the surface of the teeth to stumps, which were level with the gums. This is evident from mummies and was probably due to the high grit content of Egyptian bread, which presumably caused painful abscesses. The Ebers papyrus describes the mixing of a paste which was applied to painful gums. Some people surmise that the practice of reconstructive dentistry actually started in ancient Egypt since evidence of partial dentures or bridge work was found in a skull of about 4 500 years old. (18:49-51) The Ebers papyrus also refers to contraceptive practices including post-coital vaginal douching. (18:57,58)

Most of the treatment of disease in ancient Egypt seems to have been concentrated in the temples. These temples were part of vast complexes comprising living quarters, workshops, a school, a sacred pool and storehouses (4:120). One section was probably some sort of a clinic.

Egyptian medicine was widely respected and the Egyptians also accurately observed the stars and were skilled mathematicians. They were a pragmatic people who met the practical needs of the day. No mention is made of nursing as such, but someone must have tended the people who were treated by the priest-physicians, those with wounds, in splints, or the ill. Who they were or what exactly they did, is again a matter for conjecture. The role of *primitive mother* must have expanded to include many other people. Egyptian midwives, as a specific group of people, were however known. They formed an established, respected group of women, fulfilling a 'nursing' function.

After 1100 BCE, Egypt began to decline due to invasions by the Assyrians (663 BCE), the Persians (525 BCE), Alexander the Great (Alexandria was named after him) (332 BCE), and also by the Greeks, Romans and Muslim Arabs. Egypt did not regain its long-lost independence until 1922 CE.

1.4.5 The Cretan-Minoans

Cretan-Minoan civilisation existed on the island of Crete from about 3000 BCE until about 1400 BCE. This large island is situated in the Mediterranean Sea south of Greece, and remnants of an advanced culture with extensive systems have been excavated. The famous labyrinth of legend existed in Crete.

The art skills of the Cretan-Minoans were well developed and pottery, figurines and many well-preserved fresco paintings depict a luxurious lifestyle.

The Cretans were a seafaring nation and at one stage spread their power quite extensively. They erected massive palaces with many rooms, workshops and store-houses, as well as temples with altars (21:352). Nothing is actually known of their contribution to medicine and nursing, but such an elaborate civilisation must have had some form of health care. Like anyone else, ancient Cretans would have been subject to the ills that beset mankind.

For no apparent reason the ancient Cretan-Minoan civilisation came to an abrupt end about 1400 BCE. There is evidence of fires, but not of their cause. Again it must be pointed out that the Cretan-Minoan civilisation co-existed with other civilisations of the Ancient World (see diagram 1.1).

Diagram 1.1 Co-existence of ancient civilisations

	BCE							CE
	3500	3000	2500	2000	1500	1000	500	500
Sumerian	▬▬▬▬▬▬							
Babylonian		▬▬▬▬▬▬▬▬▬▬▬						
Assyrian				▬▬▬▬▬▬▬▬▬				
Egyptian		▬▬▬▬▬▬▬▬▬▬▬▬▬						
Cretan-Minoan			▬▬▬▬▬▬					
Persian							▬▬	
Ancient Greek					▬▬▬▬▬▬▬			
Romans								▬▬
Ancient Indian			▬▬▬▬▬▬▬▬▬▬▬▬▬▬▬▬▬					
Ancient Chinese		▬▬▬▬▬▬▬▬▬▬▬▬▬▬▬▬▬▬						
Ancient American		▬▬▬▬▬▬▬▬▬▬▬▬▬▬▬▬▬						

1.4.6 The Persians

The ancient Persian Empire was built on the former supremacy of the people known as the Medes, who probably came from southern Russia, and occupied the area today known as Iran. The actual Persian Empire only lasted about 300 years, beginning with the old Achaemedian kings, units of Iranian tribes united under Cyrus I (21:101). It existed from about 650 BCE until it was conquered by Alexander the Great in 333 BCE.

The religion of ancient Persia was based on a very old Iranian religion re-formed by Zarathustra (Greek: Zoroaster), probably around 700 BCE (32:5757). He tried to purge the ancient religion of all its gods and preached a monotheistic religious practice. He taught the application of an active form of charity, especially to the poor, kindness to animals, truthfulness and purity and the need for man to fight evil.

Avesta, the 'Scripture', are the sacred writings of the Zoroastrians, the most ancient being the Gathas which were probably composed by Zoroaster himself.

Hygienic laws seem to have been well defined, for example, spitting, blowing one's nose and eating in the street were forbidden. The pollution of rivers was prohibited, and anything that was thought to be an infectious disease was quarantined (21:118). After death, bodies were fastened to the roof of a high tower where birds picked the bones, thus preventing contamination of the earth and of rivers by decomposing bodies (8:17).

According to Lissner (21:119), medicine was a combination of magic and medical skill.

> In cases where a surgeon, a herbalist and a priest were all available, it was considered best to fetch the latter – the doctor who heals with the sacred word. Psychiatry was regarded as preferable to a surgical operation, for while there was no danger in healing the soul the scalpel could prove fatal.

Again there is no mention of nursing as such. They did however practise slavery, as slaves were exacted as tribute from subject states and certain slave-girls were listed in an inventory. The latter were obliged to dedicate their lives to the gods, presumably in temples, and no doubt also cared for the sick (21:118). The mother who traditionally cared for the children and the family undoubtedly used slaves, in the richer homes at least, for such service as well.

This civilisation seems to have been characterised by a great deal of luxury, but probably due to intermarriage the kings eventually became more and more feeble and even appear to have shown signs of mental derangement. They were eventually conquered by Alexander the Great.

1.4.7 The ancient Greeks

The classical Greek period lasted from about 1200 BCE until Greece was subjected to Roman domination in 133 BCE. Greece was not a united nation with a common capital, but consisted of numerous city states, which at times warred with one another. They spoke a common language, however, and regarded themselves as *Hellenes*, calling the land which they inhabited jointly *Hellas*. Two distinct groups of people were actually evident, that is, the *Dorians*, who were mountain folk, and the *Ionians*, who settled around the coasts. The city states started off as *monarchies* ruled by kings, followed by *oligarchies* ruled by a few people, and then *tyrannies* ruled by dictators or tyrants.

Eventually they became *democracies*, governed by the people. Among the powerful states were Sparta with a practical, hardy, conservative people, and Athens, where the inhabitants were more temperamental and imaginative. The members of these states became involved with the Ionians who had colonised the islands as well as the fringes of the mainland. Many Ionians were descendants of the ancient Mycenian culture which existed at the city of Mycenae (1600-1200 BCE), the home of Agamemnon of Trojan War fame. The tombs that have been excavated there showed among others a corpse that had apparently suffered from gallstones (1:32) and another with a fractured skull which had also been trephined. The city of Mycenae was destroyed by the Dorians when they invaded Greece.

Much of Western civilisation stems from the Greeks. Philosophy, the origin of science, evolved among these people. In pre-Hellenic Greece achievements were recorded in writings, their legends becoming epics. The art forms uncovered include sculpture, frescoes, architecture and jewellery.

The Iliad of Homer describes medical practices relating to the Trojan Wars, including the removal of foreign bodies such as arrowheads and javelins. Methods to control haemorrhage and those for the treatment of wounds are mentioned. The sun god Apollo and others were reported to 'sow infection in wounds', as well as to heal (22:49, 50).

Asklepios, who was reported to be the son of Apollo, was another deity of ancient Greece, but it is possible that he was a real person who 'became' a god after his death. Homer describes Asklepios as the 'blameless physician', and he was considered to be the god of medicine.

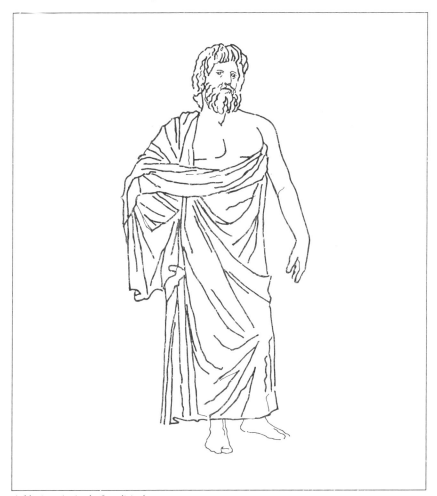

Asklepios, the 'god of medicine'

The chief seat of his worship was at Epidauros, and his cult lasted well into the Hellenic age, and was transferred to Rome in 293 BCE (32:82). He was symbolised holding a staff around which the snakes of wisdom were entwined.

This forms the basis of the present-day medical symbol, the *caduceus*. He was reputed to have had two daughters, who also came to be regarded as goddesses, namely Hygeia, the goddess of public health and Panacea, the goddess of medications. A son of Asklepios, Machaon, was described by Homer as a surgeon, serving with the Grecian force besieging Troy. Another son, Podilirius, was also an army surgeon and a psychiarist, while Telesphorus who cared for convalescents is also mentioned. Homer says that a doctor 'is worth many lives, being unequalled in removing arrows from wounds and healing them with herb ointments' (22:51).

The Asklepiades, who were supposed to be descendants of Asklepios, were an order of priests claiming a knowledge of medicine (32:82). They had to be licensed to practise medicine.

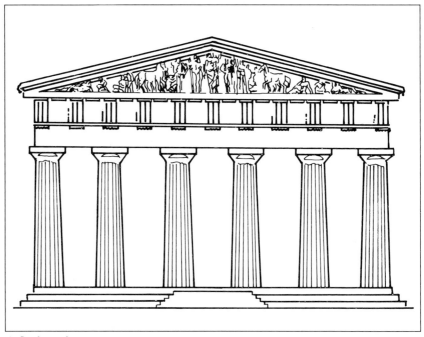

A Greek temple

The temples which were built had a sophisticated system for treating the sick and the priests of these temples were priest-physicians, interpreting dreams to decide on the appropriate form of treatment. There must have been temple attendants who assisted the priests and who must have performed nursing functions for the sick, but no reference is made to them. Massage, as part of treatment, is mentioned.

The history of the peoples of Hellenic Greece, whose influence spread to the islands and to the coast of Asia Minor, southern Italy, and Sicily is extensive. Many volumes have been devoted to their exploits. For the purpose of this book, it is only their contributions to medicine, and thus to nursing, which are mentioned.

The Hellenes were devoted to physical fitness. The Olympic Games, attended by people from a large number of city states, were held once every four years, and were celebrated in honour of the god Zeus. These games, which probably started in 776 BCE, were a tribute to the ideal of a healthy mind in a healthy body.

In the medical field the Greeks contributed to health care the need for an enquiring mind and descriptions of the treatments which were carried out at the temples.

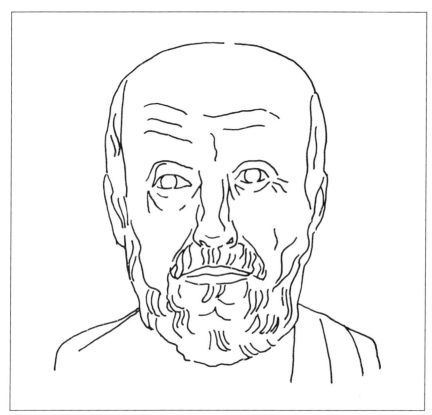

Hippocrates – the father of medicine

The work of *Hippocrates*, the so-called 'Father of Medicine' who was born on the island of Cos in 460 BCE, was of paramount importance to the development of medical care. According to Bowra (2:103), Hippocrates was 'the first and most famous of a group of physicians who formed a school of medicine in that they adhered to a common medical doctrine'. Bowra (2:104) also says that

> Hippocrates stressed the importance of careful observation and classification, and believed it was impossible to understand a part of the human body, without understanding the whole.

Hippocrates belonged to an Asklepiad family and his meticulous recording of signs and symptoms, and of successful as well as unsuccessful treatments formed the basis of scientific medicine. The idea of demon possession or a visitation of wrathful gods as a cause of disease was discarded. Hippocrates took the view that one needed to look at the whole patient, taking into account the environment from which he came, his health history and a complete physical examination. He was a great clinician and a teacher of clinical medicine. Many of the words used to describe disease conditions in Hellenic times persist in the present-day medical terminology.

Because of their careful observations, the Greeks were able to describe epidemics. They even linked the occurrence of malaria with swamps, although they did not realise the connection of malaria with mosquitoes, as ancient Indian medicine actually did. They were, however, correct in the assumption that malaria was related to marshy lands, which as we know, provides the breeding place for mosquitoes. Plague was known to have sapped the vitality of the people of Athens, but a plausible cause for the decline of the Athenian State in the fourth century BCE could well have been malaria.

In the Hippocratic period Aphrodite and Artemis were regarded as goddesses connected to fertility. The role of the priest-physician was separated from that of the midwife, whose practice was spelt out with well-defined duties.

Aphrodite was the goddess who spread life-bringing joy, and was one of the divinities who presided over the sanctity of marriage. Artemis, the twin sister of Apollo, was the goddess of the hunt. A sacrifice to Artemis was expected as part of the marriage ceremony. Artemis of Ephesus was, however, a fertility goddess, particularly venerated with Ephesus. In statues she is depicted with many breasts.

According to Shyrock (28) Hippocrates wrote about attendants of the sick in his book *On Decorum*. They were pupils of the physician who were left in charge to carry out instructions and administer treatment and watch the condition of the person being treated. These 'pupils' had to be admitted to the 'mysteries' of the art, and since women in ancient Greece were not admitted to the mysteries of any art, it can be assumed that these people, if they were actually trained attendants of the sick, were probably men.

Nurses of children, wet nurses and midwives are known to have existed. The care of the sick was probably regarded as the work of the women of the household, no doubt assisted by servants and slaves.

Medical practice became a scientific and respected calling in Hellenic times and spread throughout the known world, surviving the conquest of Greece by Macedonia, which ended when Alexander the Great died from malaria. Alexander's empire included Egypt and Alexandria, which became a famous centre of science, medicine and art, situated mainly in the university founded by Alexander on the Nile Delta. It was at Alexandria that the 'Corpus Hippocratium' was stored and where the study of human anatomy and physiology came into its own.

Hippocrates is famous for the ethical code for the practice of medicine which still forms the basis of the medical and nursing pledges of service. He may not have been the actual author of the *Hippocratic Oath* which is, however, based on his writings on ethical practice.

When Greece was captured by the Romans, Greek physicians and Greek medicine spread to all parts of this empire and thus exerted great influence on Roman medicine.

1.4.8 The ancient Romans

The civilisation of ancient Rome lasted from the legendary founding of Rome by Romulus in 753 BCE, being first ruled by Etruscan kings who were expelled by 509 BCE when the Republic was established. They ruled until 455 CE, when the Vandals sacked Rome. The last Roman Western king was expelled in 476 CE.

Before the arrival of Greek doctors in Rome, Etruscan priests seem to have served as doctors. They practised the art of divining the cause of illness by using animal organs, especially the liver. The name of soothsayer was given to the diviner. They did have some knowledge of the therapeutic properties of certain mineral waters, and also of building drains which were important for public health. The first drains were used for draining stagnant water from marshy ground, and were later adapted for sewerage (22:78).

The Etruscans also had surgeons and skilled dentists who bound teeth together with gold wire (22:79). Later the Romans also learnt the art of building aqueducts for bringing water to the cities.

The cult of Asklepios, or Aesculapius as the Romans called him, did not reach Rome until 293 BCE, but before that time 'Caesarean' section was practised to deliver the babies of women who died in childbirth (22:80).

The Roman people were materialistic and pagan. Soldiers were of value to the state, and were therefore well looked after. The Republic of Rome developed into an Empire under Caesar Augustus. Julius Caesar, who preceded him, was First Consul and later became sole ruler or dictator. It is during the time of the Roman Empire that Christ was born.

The Roman conquest spread throughout the known world, from Britain through Gaul, or France, and Spain to North Africa, including Egypt, to the Caspian Sea in the East, which included Greece, Syria, Judea, and present-day Turkey, Iraq and Iran.

Rome had two types of institutions for the care of the sick, namely, the temple and the valetudinaria. In the temple priest-physicians, assisted by temple assistants, held sway. The sick rested in the shadow of the god's temple in the hope that the god would heal them. The sick and wounded soldiers were cared for in the valetudinaria. There were also valetudinaria for sick slaves, who were regarded as valuable property. It is probable that the 'nursing' in the valetudinaria was done by slaves.

The structure of Roman life included the wealthy classes as well as the very poor. The fact is of importance later, when the contribution of the Christian Roman matrons, the female heads of Roman households, is discussed.

The Romans are well known for their administrative and legislative contribution to a civilised life. Their medical contributions are not so well known, although Hadas (13:152) points out that in Imperial Rome the rich got sick from eating and the poor from not eating, the latter falling victim to such diseases as typhoid, dysentery, diphtheria and tuberculosis. Malaria and bubonic plague also existed. Public doctors were provided for the poor from the fourth century BCE.

Hadas also states that some physicians were very sophisticated, supplying amputees with artificial limbs.

A physician who achieved fame in Rome was Asclepiades of Prusa, a Greek who had studied in Athens and Alexandria before coming to Rome in 91 BCE. He was a fashionable doctor who prescribed diet and exercise, including walking, baths and massage.

Aulus Aurelius Cornelius Celsus (25 BCE – 50 CE) wrote *De Medicina* which consisted of eight books. Books I and II deal principally with diet, principles of therapeutics and pathology, III and IV with internal diseases and V and VI with external diseases and pharmaceutical preparations, while VII and VIII deal with diseases calling for surgical treatment (32:1135). Among others he described nutrient enemas, plastic surgery on the nose, lips and ears, the care of wounds, the typing of blood vessels and the suturing of wounds. He used the well-known terms, *rubor* – redness, *calor* – heat, *dolor* – pain, *tumor* – swelling, which have become the classic terms for describing inflammation. He also described treatment for fractures and abdominal surgery. Among the surgical instruments of his time which have been found are forceps, scalpels, clips, probes and tongs. It is interesting when one realises that although this work was written almost 2000 years ago, it still sounds familiar to nurses and doctors of the late 20th century.

The conquests of foreign lands were responsible for diseases spreading to all parts of the empire. It has been suggested that the decline of the Roman empire was due, partially at least, to the lead piping which they used to carry water and to the practice of storing wine in lead vats, drinking acidic wine from lead cups and cooking in pots made of lead, all of which probably caused extensive lead poisoning.

Bones uncovered in a Roman cemetery of about the 4th and 5th centuries showed concentrations of lead much higher than normal. Lead is also known to lead to infertility which may also have contributed to the fall of Rome (18:191).

The Romans built valetudinaria throughout their empire for the care of their sick and wounded soldiers. The first hospitals were simple structures built around courtyards, with provision made for latrines and baths. There were separate wards connected by a corridor. By the end of the 4th century CE hospitals were based on the military example of providing places where the sick could be cared for in places outside the home, a practice which found much favour among the Christians. After the fall of the Roman Empire the valetudinaria were abandoned and much of what had been was lost (18:187).

In Roman times the skill of the midwife was of paramount importance in childbirth. Margotta (22:88) states that parturition is a normal physiological process which does not on the whole need medical intervention; thus the role of the doctor has always been minor. Abnormal positions of the foetus were recognised as being likely causes of difficulties in childbirth. The work of the Roman Soranus, which was concerned with gynaecology and related subjects, will be discussed later among the prominent people of the Christian Era.

1.4.9 The ancient Israelites

This group of ancient people who continue to exist as the Jews of today, made a great contribution to medical and hygienic practices. The accounts of their origin are contained in the early books of the Bible. They probably migrated from Haran in Mesopotamia to Canaan, later Palestine, and now Israel. They lived a pastoral life in Canaan until they were forced by famine to migrate to Egypt, where they got permission to settle in Goshen. There they flourished until they were later subjected to repressive measures. About 1304-1237 BCE Moses led them out of Egypt, back towards Canaan, 'the promised land' (32:2957).

The Israelites underwent many vicissitudes, being conquered by various peoples throughout the ages. Yet they preserved their identity and their religion. In Exodus 15:26 the Lord said to Moses: 'If you listen to the voice of the Lord and pay attention to his commands . . . I will not bring on you any of the diseases I brought on the Egyptians, for I am the Lord who heals you' (17). The ancient Israelites were thus told that health was theirs if they followed the commands of the Lord.

In *An illustrated history* Margotta (22:35) states the following.

> For the ancient Hebrews, disease was not due to a demon, or evil spirit, or to spells cast by jealous men, but represented a visible sign of God's wrath at the sins of men. Health could never fail as long as the Ten Commandments were observed . . . priests were arbiters of the law of Moses, and did more health work than doctors.

The Mosiac Code of laws is an outstanding example of a systematic prescription for healthy living and the prevention of disease. The following excerpts are taken from the *New international version of the Bible*, and give an idea of some of the health 'laws' laid down.

The book of Leviticus describes regulations for the management of persons with any infectious skin disease, for an itch, for mildew in clothing or in a house, and for a swelling, rash or a bright spot. It describes isolation for persons with infectious diseases and for cleansing on recovery. Clear distinction is made between what can be regarded as 'clean', and what 'unclean'. Chapter 15 discusses measures to be taken when

□ a man has a bodily discharge, as well as the care of clothes of the sufferer, and the precautions anyone must take who touches the man, his clothing etc

□ a man has an emission of semen

□ a woman menstruates, describing menstrual hygiene

□ a woman has a discharge other than the menstrual flow.

Personal hygiene, especially regarding rest, diet, sleep, cleanliness and working hours was emphasised. Meticulous description of the care of the hands and clothing is given. Chapter 17 forbids the eating of blood and says that an animal may be eaten only after the blood has been drained. Deuteronomy 23:12-13 describes what had to be done in camps regarding human excreta, the individual being required to go out of camp, dig a hole and cover the excrement afterwards.

The high-priest was both a priest physician and a health inspector. The Hebrews believed that visiting and caring for the sick was a religious duty.

Although it does not form part of the Mosiac health code, Genesis 17:12 decrees that every male child be circumcised at the age of eight days.

Margotta (22:36) also stated that 'when an epidemic was waging the alarm was sounded on the shofar (or ram's horn)' and that some of the rules about food were based on specific medical observation. He further states that Hebrew surgeons were very skilful, performing operations for anal fistula and imperforate ani in the newborn. They also undertook Caesarean section and treated fractures and dislocations by using rational measures.

According to Margotta (22:36) the Talmud also contains accurate information about anatomy and physiology and the description of diseases such as jaundice, cirrhosis of the liver, parasitic diseases, diphtheria and even haemophilia.

Midwifery was an established practice among the Israelites and midwives held an honoured place in the community. Exodus 1:15 states that the King of Egypt 'spoke to the Hebrew midwives'. Delivery stools are also mentioned in this chapter, while Ezekiel 16:4 mentions Hebrew birth practices such as cutting the cord, washing the baby with water to clean it, rubbing the child with salt and wrapping it in cloth. The ethical code of midwives is stated regarding the preservation of life. The Hebrew contribution to the care of the sick, although considerable, was more concerned with prophylaxis than treatment. Nurses, besides midwives, are mentioned, Deborah being the first to be recorded in the 24th chapter of Genesis.

It was the duty of early Hebrew priests to recognise lepers and isolate them from the community. Although it is probable that other diseases were mistaken for leprosy, this was a form of community health practice (28:164).

In the course of time the priests built up an empirical knowledge of the effects of different kinds of baths, ointments and poultices, which they made from herbs and oils on various skin conditions, abscesses and the like. They were thus a kind of priest physician and probably passed their knowledge on to 'lay' students, leading to the development of lay healers or 'doctors'.

Jewish healers made up medications from powdered roots or by soaking berries or leaves in water and giving the concoctions to 'patients' to drink.

They also practised surgery but could not study anatomy because their religion forbade them to dissect dead bodies. Examples of tools used by Jewish healers, probably influenced by Romans, have been found and include scalpels, retractors, probes and hooks for various purposes (including the scraping away of tissue and a box for medicines). These tools were found in various places during the excavation of old sites in Israel, including Masada.

The Israeli city of Jericho is the oldest city known to mankind for its medications, notably the sap from its balsam trees, which reputedly cured headaches and was also used to 'treat cataracts' (18:44).

This remarkable people still practise the health laws laid down so many centuries ago. Theirs is the only major religion which does not have elaborate churches and temples. Their synagogues are relatively simple and are places of worship, not built to glorify a god or gods.

1.4.10 Ancient India

In the study of health care in ancient civilisations the reader of the late 20th century of the Christian or Common Era must pause to think. With jet air travel, radio communication and television with satellite transmission, communication is so easy that reports of happenings in far parts of the world are conveyed almost instantaneously.

The idea of civilisations developing at the same period of time, yet having no knowledge of each other's existence, is almost unthinkable. Yet communication took a considerable time as voyages by sea in small boats or overland travel using animals as the most rapid means of propulsion meant very long, often tedious and dangerous journeys. Messages could be sent only by beating drums or perhaps smoke signals. Even pigeon post was a much later development.

If all this is borne in mind, and a perspective is kept of parallel growth of various civilisations, then it will be easier for the modern student to appreciate the remarkable health care practised by ancient peoples in isolation from one another.

Records of civilisations in Ancient India exist from 2500 BCE when the Indus Valley civilisation flourished. India was cut off from the Western World by high mountains and vast seas. North-eastern India was invaded about 1500 BCE and this civilisation flourished until Darius of Persia conquered the people of that time. Eventually Alexander the Great reached India.

The history of India was chequered, but it extended until 1700 CE when the Mugdal empire collapsed. Later conquests, including that of the British, and eventual independence fall outside the scope of this chapter once more.

Since the fourth century BCE the religion of India was Hinduism and later, after about 552 BCE when Buddha ('the enlightened one') was born, Buddhism also gained prominence. The gods of ancient India were ferocious and were served by a separate priesthood who performed sacrificial rituals.

The sacred 'Books of Learning', the Veda, were produced in the Vedic period from 1500 BCE. The Ayurveda (the Veda of Long Life) was particularly concerned with medicine, and describes medical treatment by the use of incantation (22:30).

Indian medicine flourished under two prominent Indian doctors, Charaka and Susruta. Though they lived in the Christian Era, their work will be discussed here, as they were not influenced by Christianity at all. Charaka, who lived in the second century after the birth of Christ, wrote eight books mainly devoted to medicine whilst Susruta, who lived in the fourth century AD, wrote six, which contain a fair knowledge of human anatomy and are mainly concerned with surgery.

Indian surgeons were skilled in a wide range of operations, including tonsillectomy, lithotomy, incision of abscesses and amputations. They seem to have been particularly good at reshaping the nose,which was frequently cut off as a punishment for some crime. This meant that they actually practised an early form of plastic surgery. Earlobes were also replaced by plastic surgery.

According to Margotta (22:34) the instruments known to ancient Indian surgeons included scalpels, saws, scissors, forceps for tooth extraction and for removing foreign bodies from ears, probes, catheters, needles for suturing and even syringes. Further, he also states that their diagnostic technique was of a relatively high standard, and included inspection, palpation and auscultation.

Psychosomatic cause of illness was understood, and accurate descriptions of diabetes mellitus, tuberculosis and smallpox are found. Indian medicine also related malaria to mosquitoes, and plague to rodents. Treatment included purgatives, enemas, emetics, the application of leeches, steam baths and inhalations.

Margotta (22:34) states that Susruta lists 760 medical plants which include *Atropa belladonna* and *Cannibis indica,* and *Rauwolfia serpentina* which was used for sedation.

Susruta believed that the physician, the patient, the medicine and the attendants are the four essential factors of a course of medical treatment. Although no mention is made of nurses as such, with the exception of the attendants of Susruta, the nature of treatments, including the care of people who underwent surgery, must have required some skills other than those of the surgeons. Who gave this care is not clear, but it was surely a form of nursing care that was given by 'attendants' or others.

Hinduism laid down very strict hygiene rules, such as a vegetarian diet, no alcohol, emphasis on cleanliness and bathing and the immediate removal of excreta and other waste matter from the house.

1.4.11 Ancient China

William Watson (24:267) states that the history of China is in the main the history of a single people using a single language and a system of writing that has not changed in principle from its beginning over 3 000 years ago. Margotta (22:41) writes that 'while the pharaohs of Egypt were engrossed in erecting pyramids, the ancient Chinese emperors were preoccupied with medicine'.

Shen Nung, who is thought to have ruled from 2838 to 2698 BCE, compiled three volumes on herbs which list 365 herbs, prescriptions and poisons. Drugs mentioned in these writings which are not unfamiliar in the 1990s include the use of opium as a narcotic, rhubarb as a laxative, flowers of Artemisia for worms, Rauwolfia as a sedative, kaolin for diarrhoea, ephedrine for asthma and chaulmoogra oil for leprosy. Other drugs used in ancient China are sodium sulphate for purging, iron for anaemia and arsenic for skin disorders.

They are also known to be the first to immunise against smallpox (22:42).

Diagnostic examination was apparently not understood, but surgery was practised, sometimes even using primitive narcotics and anaesthesia. The practice of medicine was taught at a medical college which was controlled by the emperors of China, who also introduced state examinations (22:46).

Schafer (25:130) also mentions the use of 'iodine-rich seaweeds to treat goitre and ergot, a rye fungus, to alleviate uterine difficulties during childbirth'. According to him the ancient Chinese contracted beri-beri from eating only polished rice. This was treated by the use of a gourd drink which supplied the missing vitamin, while liver and kidneys of pigs and the eyes of sheep were used and were actually an empirical prevention of other vitamin deficiencies.

Schafer says further that 'the early study of medicine was sanctified by the belief that the ancient holy shamans (medicine men or priest-physicians) had the power to heal both the body and the mind'. He also states that by the sixth century BCE secular physicians with no shamanistic powers had come into being, while by the third century BCE, physicians had specialised into various fields. Thus there were specialists such as dieticians, veterinarians and specialists in internal and external medicine. Acupuncture, a common practice in those days, is still used today.

Although no mention is made of nurses, a painting dating as far back as 1200 BCE shows a village doctor applying treatment, accompanied by a doctor's *assistant*. It is interesting to note what an advanced medical system evolved ahead of or concurrently with what was occurring in other parts of the world, and yet quite independently.

1.4.12 The African continent

This continent and its early history has only been the subject of intensive study over the last century, although early travellers reported sighting some cities such as Timbuktu and there is some evidence of civilisations on the central continent. It seems, however, that up to about 500 BCE people south of the Sahara lived in Stone Age simplicity (7:21).

The civilisations around the Nile Valley and Egypt have been described generally in section 1.4.4. As yet there is no evidence of ancient civilisations south of Zimbabwe, so that knowledge of medicine and its sister profession, nursing, in those areas is not available either.

However, the southern tip of Africa was populated by primitive peoples who had some form of social organisation into tribes and as their way of life has remained practically unchanged for many, many centuries, some knowledge of their medical practices may be gleaned from present-day rituals. The 'medicine men', for example, have endured as a group into this century and must have filled an important part in tribal life and early medical care. Primitive mother, in her extended sphere, must also have filled her caring role in whatever 'civilisation' existed.

There appears to have been a large body of empirical knowledge among the tribes, much of which was passed down to the present day. Various rites were carried out to cast out evil spirits which were thought to be the cause of illnesses. These included chanting, pummeling the body (the origin of massage?), the casting out of evil spirits and the use of various charms. Sometimes a hideous mask was worn by the 'medicine man' to frighten off the evil spirits. Ritual dancing was also used as part of the treatment. The human body within which the evil spirit was harboured, had to be transformed into an unpleasant place for the spirit. Herbs which could cause vomiting or purging would be used to rid the body of these unwanted 'visitors'.

Various types of traditional healers, including the *wise women* of the tribe came into existence. These wise women seem to have become quite skilled in the use of herbs, many of which were very effective.

In an unpublished study on traditional and modern approaches to the health care of pregnant women in Xhosa society (3:44) Baartman has made some interesting observations including

☐ appealing to ancestors for their favour and assistance

☐ frequent warm water massage of the sides by the traditional birth attendant in prolonged labour

☐ cutting of the cord by a thick stalk of tambookie-grass

☐ giving the woman who has difficulty in labour an infusion of a horse's placenta to drink.

Harper (15:408) is quoted as saying that 'it contains large amounts of the hormone *relaxin* [which] has the ability to bring about the relaxation of the symphysis pubis'. He also discusses the traditional methods of dealing with the placenta and the cord, as well as other customs related to childbirth, the nuerperium and the care of the baby.

1.4.13 Ancient America

At the far side of the globe different civilisations developed in the Americas, especially in the present-day Mexico and Peru. It appears as if *Homo sapiens* evolved in the 'Old World', that is Europe and Asia, also migrating in small numbers from eastern Siberia, the Bering Strait and Alaska (20:11,12), probably bringing cultural equipment such as clothing, means of shelter and tools with him.

By 2000 BCE agriculture had become a way of life in Middle America (20:17), and a diversity of peoples dwelt in the varied lands of ancient America. These people left a vivid record of themselves and their civilisations in the wealth of sculptured figures unearthed by archaeologists (20:19).

Temples and cities have been unearthed depicting priests making sacrifices to gods. The magic rite of attempted transference of disease to animals seems to have been practised (8:36). Apparently emetics, laxatives and diuretics as well as various poisons were known.

Ancient civilisations were those of the Olmecs, along Mexico's Gulf coast, the Maya of southern Mexico and Central America, and the Aztecs, whose empire spread into Peru, Argentina, Bolivia and Chile. Early civilisations in Peru had many artefacts. One of particular interest to students of health care is a seated Mochican cripple with a stump for a leg, carrying a heavy staff.

The cult of a jaguar god, a man-jaguar, was practised in Peru after 1000 BCE. Ambitious local medicine men won additional power by becoming priests of the new faith (20:81). Evidence also exists of a great deal of war-like activity, which would have brought with it its toll of injuries, which meant that people required health care and attention. Captured peoples were enslaved and class distinction is clearly depicted.

> Like most primitive people, the early inhabitants of Middle America appear to have worshipped simple nature deities, such as the sun and the moon, and the gods of rain, springtime and fertility. Sometimes mountains and trees were held sacred and corn was the sacred plant (20:103).

Later sterner gods were worshipped who 'demanded' human sacrifice. Adult human hearts and children were sacrificed by different groups. Mummified bodies, wrapped in magnificent cloth, have been found dating from early civilisations.

The elaborate civilisations of ancient America appear to have had no written language; thus word of mouth served as their only communication medium. However, the Aztecs appear to have had a kind of hieroglyphic writing (20:33).

Dolan (8:33) points out that skull deformation,which started four to five days after birth, was common among the Mayas. One apparent medical practice was the use of sweat baths, as well as trephining.

Dolan (8:35,36) also notes that a pottery or stone effigy of the sick person was made which, together with skeletal remains, have left a record of pathological conditions which existed in ancient America. The squatting position was normally used for delivering babies, as can be seen in many clay figurines.

1.5 Conclusion

A review of primitive cultures and medical practices reveals that the care of sick people was practised in some form, and that many practices had a remarkable similarity despite the fact that the people who used them existed far apart and even at widely differing periods in the history of the planet earth. Researchers have also shown that many diseases which are known today were found in the early inhabitants of the surface of the globe.

Civilisations waxed and waned, customs and beliefs also underwent change and different social types which varied to meet the needs of place and time, arose. *Homo sapiens*, with his adaptable nature, has survived despite disease and injury. He has been born, grown to maturity and, in many cases, reached a fairly advanced age. Of course there have been unwanted deaths among the young, and even human sacrifice. At birth man is one of the most helpless of creatures, unable to survive for several years without nurturing, that is 'nursing', and *primitive mother* must have been the first to give that care. Many medical practices have been revealed by the study of ancient civilisations, some of which were quite sophisticated.

People with fractured limbs in splints must have needed care too, and some person had to provide that care. That person was probably a mother, a surrogate mother or a member of the extended family. Neighbours, temple attendants, slaves or other people to whom such tasks were designated, were giving health care to those in need of such care. It can be stated, without fear of contradiction, that they were *nursing* as it was practised in the time in which they lived.

During a recent visit to Greece including Crete, Turkey and Israel, the author was struck by the use that was made of water as a purifying agent in the ancient civilisations of those parts of the world. Water must have been a very precious commodity in those hot climates, and springs and fresh water were no doubt precious. The Greeks washed in these waters before entering the temples of the Gods and the ritual purification bath of the Hebrews, the 'mikvah', exists to this day among traditional Jews.

2

THE DAWN OF THE CHRISTIAN ERA

Jesus Christ or Jesus 'The Anointed One' was born during the reign of Caesar Augustus, at Bethlehem in Judaea, a Roman province at that time. Mary, his mother, and Joseph, his foster father, had to flee to Egypt because of threats made by Herod (73 BCE-4 CE), who was appointed governor of Galilee by Anthony in 40 BCE. On Herod's death Mary and Joseph returned to their home town of Nazareth (present-day Al-Nasira) where Christ grew to manhood, quietly pursuing Joseph's trade of carpentry. At the age of about 30 he started his brief ministry which lasted between one and three years, and consisted of public preaching and private instruction of his disciples. Closely connected with Christ's teaching was his ministry of healing, with which this work is mainly concerned (32:3055, 3056).

The advent of Christ and of Christianity had a profound effect on the attitude of people to the sick and the suffering. After Christ's death on the cross, his teaching and philosophy were carried to many parts of the world, first by his original disciples and then by those converted to Christianity. Paul and Barnabas, neither of whom were one of the original 12 disciples, spread the teachings of Christianity to Asia Minor.

At first Christians were persecuted and martyred. This persecution reached its greatest severity under Caius Valerius Diocletianus, or the emperor Diocletian, around the year 303 CE. However, the persecution only served to strengthen the 'new' religion and the Christian church eventually received official recognition under the emperor Constantine in about 313 CE, although Constantine did not actually become a Christian until he was on his deathbed in 337 CE. In 326 CE Constantine moved the capital of the Roman Empire from Rome to Byzantium, which he renamed Constantinople. Christianity became the official religion of the state during the reign of Theodosius the Great (379-395 CE). St Luke was a Greek physician, a Gentile of Antioch, who is credited with having written the third gospel. He was closely associated with the work of St Paul, by whom he was called 'the beloved physician'.

There are some famous people, non-Christians, who achieved distinction during the Christian Era. They were born and lived and worked during the time when Christianity was spreading and Christians were beginning to practise their religion publicly. Some of the early Christians will be discussed in the following section.

2.1 Famous medical names in the early Christian era

This section only gives the names of those people who became famous during this time, together with a brief résumé of their achievements. They are selected not only for their fame but also for their scientific approach to medicine, which must have had an effect on those who provided *nursing* care to the patients.

☐ *Aulus Cornelius Celsus* (25 BCE-50 CE) has already been mentioned in section 1.4.8.

☐ *Caius Plinius Secundus* (23-79 CE) was known as Pliny the elder. He produced an encyclopaedic work of 37 volumes which include many references to animal, vegetable and mineral drugs, as well as to public-health measures. He died after the disastrous eruption of Vesuvius (22:86, 87).

☐ *Soranus of Ephesus* lived in the first century of the Christian Era and was the most famous obstetrician of ancient times. He described the extraction of the foetus by the use of forceps or hooks to deliver a baby who could not be born normally, as well as methods which could be employed to reduce abnormal positions of the foetus by external manipulation, so as to effect the eventual normal delivery of a child. Soranus was also interested in such aspects as breastfeeding, weaning, teething and the general care of the newborn baby and young child.

☐ *Pedanius Dioscorides* (40-90 CE) was a Greek physician who served with the Roman armies. His claim to fame is the production of the five books, known as *De Materia Medica*. These books not only gave us the term *materia medica*, which is still in use in the 20th century, but were also original works in the field. The use of herbs, ointments, animal products, plants and roots, wines, and minerals such as lead acetate, copper oxide and calcium hydroxide for medical purposes were described in them.

☐ *Claudius Galen* (130-203 CE) was the most famous of ancient doctors and his name is remembered to this day. He was extremely well known both as a practising physician and as a writer, producing about 400 medical disser-tations. He studied anatomy mainly through the dissection of animals, which gave him a distorted picture of the anatomy of the human body. He also conducted experiments on animals to study physiology. According to Margotta (22:96) 'he declared that every alteration in function resulted from an organic lesion and conversely that every organic lesion led to alteration of function. This concept remains substantially valid.'

Galen was not a Christian, but it appears that he believed in one god, and he was thus acceptable to the early Christian church as well as to the Hebrews and Arabs. He was a skilled diagnostician and Galen has been credited with being the first occupational health physician because of his description of diseases specific to those working in mines.

☐ *Cosmas* and *Damian* were twin brothers who were martyred by the emperor Diocletian and thus, strictly speaking, do not fall into the group of non-Christian medical men. Arabs by birth, they practised medicine in

Asia Minor and were actually the first two Christian doctors who practised healing by the use of faith.

2.2 The deaconesses

In the early Christian church women, known as deaconesses, worked among the sick. They were in fact the first known official visiting nurses and carried out Christian acts of caring for the sick, giving water to the thirsty, feeding the hungry, and clothing the naked. The aim of their actions was to practise Christian compassion and to give spiritual support to those in need, such as prisoners and the homeless, and where necessary to bury the dead. However, their primary duty was to assist at the baptism of women, and to minister to sick and needy women.

Before the advent of women dedicated to caring for the suffering, such as deaconesses, nursing care was part of the extended role of the mother, as existed in primitive societies, or was given by slaves. As this was not their chosen work, but was forced on them by circumstance, the loving care provided by women to whom it was a religious duty, was missing from the care provided by slaves.

The first known deaconess was Phoebe of Cenchrea, who was mentioned by St Paul, the apostle, in his epistle to the Romans in chapter 16:1-2, circa 58 CE:

> I commend to you our sister Phoebe, a servant [or deaconess – 17:205] of the church in Cenchrea. I ask you to receive her in the Lord in a way worthy of the saints and to give her any help she may need from you, for she has been of great help to many people including me.

Phoebe was a rich woman who travelled extensively and was thus able to spread her influence wherever she went. Deaconesses are also mentioned by St Paul in his epistle to Timothy.

St John Chrysostom (345-407 CE), one of the so-called 'fathers of the church' who became Patriarch of Constantinople (although later exiled), also described Olympias, a rich woman of his time, as a deaconess. A young widow who was born in 368 CE, Olympias founded a house of deaconesses, whose inmates devoted themselves to works of Christian *charity* (today translated as *'love'*) and caring for the sick and needy. It was an ascetic order, the members of which neglected themselves and their bodies as an offering to God.

Other well-known deaconesses of the early church were Praxides and Pudentiana, who are especially known for their work among prisoners.

Little has been written about the life of deaconesses, but it is known that they were the only order of women who were ordained by the *'laying on of hands'*. The order of deaconesses was established and became important in early church work, but gradually faded into insignificance. In the Western World the work of deaconesses was probably supplanted by that of the religious sisters, as the church moved towards monasticism. Their existence as a separate group continued for much longer in the church of the Eastern part of the world.

Deaconesses, as special female workers for the church, have been revived by the Reformed churches in recent times.

2.3 The Roman matrons

The spreading of Christianity in the Roman empire of the day resulted in changed attitudes towards the care of the sick and needy. Among the Roman women who devoted themselves to this act of love, were several so-called 'Roman matrons'. They were wealthy Roman women who were converted to Christianity and sought to practise their new faith by ministering to the sick, the disabled and the poor. Many of them were responsible for the building of early Christian hospitals.

☐ *Helena* (c 250-330 CE), one of the most famous of the Roman matrons, was a Roman empress and the mother of the emperor Constantine. She became a Christian after the Edict of Milan in 313 CE and made a pilgrimage to Palestine to visit holy places. She is remembered for having founded the first Christian hospital in Jerusalem (36:4).

☐ *Flacilla* was the wife of the emperor Theodosius. She attended to the needs of the sick in hospital and was particularly interested in those with physical handicaps (8:69).

☐ *Marcella*, a rich woman renowned for her scholarship, was inspired by St Jerome to convert her luxurious palace in Rome into a convent where women were taught the care of the sick. She could thus be described as the first nurse-educator (8:69).

☐ *Fabiola,* also a disciple of St Jerome, is credited with building the first hospital in the Western World, in Rome, in 390 CE (22:102). St Basil built the first big Christian hospital at Caesarea in present-day Israel (28 km from Tel-Aviv): 'It had as many wards as there were diseases to treat and resembled a little township on its own; it included a leper colony.' (22:102).

Before the actual building of hospitals as such, those pilgrims who became sick on the way were cared for in hospices or *xenodochia,* which served as shelters for pilgrims to the holy land. Other places of care for the sick in Roman times were known as *nosocomia,* 'houses of the sick', and *gerokomia,* 'houses of the aged'.

The well-known painting of Fabiola by JJ Henner (1829-1905) is an artist's impression, and not from real life. It has been taken as symbolising the Roman matrons, who were so justly famous in the early Christian Era.

☐ *Paula* (347-404 CE), another noble Roman matron of the period, joined St Jerome with other members of the Roman community in Antioch, eventually settling in Bethlehem in 386 CE. Paula established three convents, and she and her followers devoted themselves to a life of asceticism and study (32:3032). She also played a role in building a hospital in Bethlehem where she and the sisters of the community nursed the sick and the poor in the only way that was known to them, that is, by washing, feeding and making them comfortable and supporting those who were dying with spiritual comfort.

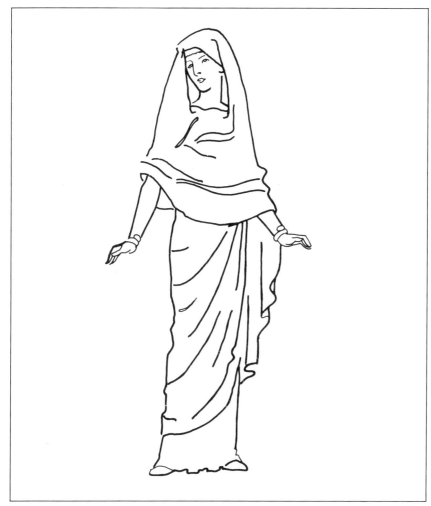

An impression of Fabiola

2.4 The Paraboloni

The Paraboloni were a group of Christian men, 'brothers in Christ', who were reputed to have banded together during the great plague of Alexandria, in the second half of the third century of the Christian Era. The first Christian monks thus came from Egypt (8:71, 72)

The Paraboloni were dedicated to caring for the sick, comforting the dying, burying the dead and considered it to be their Christian duty to clean out infected houses. They also acted as health visitors. This group is important to nursing history because they were an order of men caring for the sick, that is they are the first known male nurses.

2.5 General aspects of Christian health care

The Christian religion taught compassion for those less fortunate than oneself. There was, however, an ambivalent attitude to suffering (1:4). The early Christians believed that this life was transitory and that any personal suffering was to be borne with patience, as a 'purification' for the life hereafter. This attitude tended to stifle any enquiry into the cause of disease. Dissection of human bodies was frowned on as the body was regarded as God's temple, and as such not to be violated, even after death. Medical care — and thus nursing care too — was an act of Christian love which all members of the community were expected to carry out as their bounden duty. Thus it cannot be said that Christianity did much to enhance medical knowledge.

With the decline of the Roman Empire many terrible epidemics and plagues swept through the empire. Man, knowing nothing of micro-organisms and methods of disease prevention, was powerless. These epidemics caused much harm to the improvement of medical knowledge as it appeared to the people of the period that bodily ills could only be treated by divine intervention, and the practice of 'faith healing' (22:101, 102).

Christianity cherished the belief that 'all people were worthy of being loved and cared for . . . the concept of the brotherhood of man' (34:4).

Although early Christian hospitals owed much to the charitable work of prominent women, they were also the concern of the leaders in the church, the bishops.

According to Donahue (9:117) rooms in houses for the care of the sick, poor and aged were established fairly early and known as *diakonia*. They soon became too small and had to have additions made. Whole new buildings were built, which housed all unfortunates needing charitable care — these became known as *xenodochia* and were financed by the church and run by deaconesses.

A famous *xenodochium* was founded by St Basil in Caesarea in 370 CE and provided hospital care, preventive care and social service (9:121, 122). It had resident nurses and specialised sections, including a section for the care of lepers and other contagious diseases, a section for the aged and another for the insane. By this monasteries became more than just a place for prayer and ascetic practices, and provided not only medical treatment for the sick, but also relief for the poor (9:207).

Little is known of the nursing care given as such, or about any form of formal or informal training of those attending to the sick, although orders of religious nursing sisters grew up within the church, some of which exist to this very day.

Monasteries usually had infirmaries for the sick and a herb garden where herbs were grown. Sometimes these were special 'physic' gardens.

Francis of Assisi (CE 1118-1226) was another Christian whose order cared for the sick in their homes (9:263)

2.6 Arabic learning

Islam, the religion preached by Mohammed, purported to revive the faith that was taught first to Adam and then to Abraham (32:2952). Mohammed (really Muhammed — 'praised' or 'praiseworthy') was born in Mecca (date unknown) and died in 632 CE. Thus he lived in the sixth and seventh century of the early Christian Era.

The Arab world which Mohammed was to wield together 'was in contact with the older civilisations and had access to the collected Greek writings in the library of Alexandria, and for a few centuries after the death of . . . Mohammed . . . led the world in medical teaching' (1:4, 5).

The Islamic religion taught men to enquire into the reasons for illness and death, with the result that medical knowledge made vast progress.

Only two famous Arabic medical writers will be discussed here, as the others fall into a later period.

☐ *Rhazes* (Abu Bakr Muhammed Ibn Zakariyah Al-Razi, 850-923 CE) wrote 117 medical books in which he meticulously described smallpox, chicken pox and measles, based on his own direct observation, experience and conclusions. He also devoted an entire treatise to the diseases of children. He was originally a Persian from near Teheran, and studied medicine at Baghdad (32:4630).

☐ *Avicenna* (Ibn Sina, 980-1037 CE) was the author of the famous text *Canon of Medicine* (Al-Quanam) in which he attempted to codify all known medical knowledge (32:425). His most important medical works were the *Al-Hawi* or *Continens*, an encyclopaedia of medicine, and the *Liber Almansoris*, which was compiled from various earlier writers and showed how completely Greek medicine was transmitted to Arabic medicine.

The Arabs also organised a hospital system where patients were nursed by male and female attendants under the supervision of a physician. The hospitals were divided into different sections to cope with different types of disease, and included an outpatient department where medicines were distributed to those not admitted to hospital. Treatment was apparently free, and some attempt seems to have been made for the training of doctors (1:5).

3

THE MIDDLE AGES

The period known as the *Middle Ages* is usually taken to cover the thousand years from the death of Constantine I in 337 CE, to about 1453 CE, with the fall of Constantinople (modern Istanbul) to the Turks. It is the intermediate period between the culture of classical antiquity and the Renaissance (32:3681).

Because the period was not one of continuous progress, it will be considered in two sections, and the nursing implications will be highlighted wherever possible.

3.1 The Medieval period or early Middle Ages (337-1200 CE)

This period is also known as the Dark Ages, for barbarian invaders destroyed much of Roman civilisation with the fall of Rome in 476 CE. Despite the prevailing disorganisation and disorder, Christianity survived but medieval knowledge of physical science was negligible and education on the whole conservative (32:3681).

The majority of people of that period were poor farmers, known as *serfs*, who lived a hand to mouth existence under primitive conditions. Life was hard and life expectancy short.

The nobility or upper class were mainly a warlike group of people who ruled their particular areas and to whom the serfs owed allegiance, in return for which they received a certain amount of protection from marauding tribes.

The third group of people of the times were those concerned with the religious organisations, namely, the priests. These men, who were to be found in the monasteries, as well as in the community at large, were bound by their religious vows and subject to the control of the hierarchy of the church, with the supreme bishop being the Bishop of Rome or the Pope.

3.1.1 Christian monasticism

Christian monasticism, founded in the early days of the Christian church, spread rapidly during this period. It was responsible for keeping alive what learning there was and expanded to include educational and artistic pursuits. St Benedict (480-547 CE), who was born at Nursia in Italy, founded the celebrated monastery at Montecassino in 529 CE. The Benedictine Order attracted the most followers and is still very active (32:3756).

St Benedict felt that the care of the sick should be placed above and before every other duty and that Christ was directly served by waiting on the sick (1:79). To this end monks cultivated herbs for the treatment of the sick and, because of the care given there, the monasteries became the centres for medical education.

An order of *oblates*, not monks or nuns but laymen and laywomen dedicated to God and to his service, was also formed, attached to the Benedictine monastery. Other orders of oblates were also established. Thus organised care of the sick by the laity was also practised in this period.

3.1.2 Nursing saints

The status of women in the general population was inferior, but there was an acknowledged place for them in religious communities, where they could rise to powerful positions in convents as abbesses and the like.

Religious sisters or nuns, women who dedicated their lives to the service of God were active in many fields, among which were teaching and nursing. Some, whose main sphere of activity was nursing, became famous for their exemplary lives and service to suffering humanity and were eventually canonised by the church. These wonderful women are known as nursing saints and include:

☐ *Brigit of Kildare* (450-525 CE), also known as Brigid or Bridget, founded the first nunnery in Ireland, at Kildare (32:832). She not only instituted higher learning for women, but also tended the sick, particularly lepers, together with her nuns (1:80).

☐ *Scholastica* (480-? CE), the twin sister of Benedict, founded a community for women near Montecassino, where the nuns attended the sick and needy. She is buried in the monastery of Montecassino.

☐ *Radegunde* (518-587 CE), a Frankish queen, was converted to Christianity. She left her husband because of his disgusting behaviour, which included ill-treatment and murder, to become a nun. She later founded the nunnery of Holy Cross at Poitiers (32:4532) where sisters devoted themselves to the care of the sick and to study. She also built a hospital in which special care was given to lepers (1:81).

☐ *Clothilde* or *Clothilda* (475-545 CE), was also a Frankish queen, who came from a Christian background and later converted her husband. After his death she retired to the abbey of St Martin at Tours where she performed what she regarded as her Christian duty, namely caring for the sick (32:1338).

The following laywomen, engaged in the care of the sick and the alleviation of suffering, were canonised by the Church. Women such as these expanded the effects of Christianity by providing care of the sick as part of what they believed to be their Christian duty.

☐ *Margaret* (1045-1093), a deeply religious Scottish queen, gave money to the poor, visited hospitals and helped to tend the sick (32:3535).

☐ *Dymphna* (early sixth century CE) was a young Irish princess who according to legend ran away from her crazed father and was murdered in the forests of Geel near Antwerp in Belgium. Those who visited her tomb were reported to have been miraculously cured and a shrine was eventually built there. It soon became a place where the mentally ill and retarded were cared for and psychiatric care is still available in the colony that grew up around this shrine.

Although people in the Middle Ages lived very isolated lives, medieval Europe was spiritually a commonwealth, a quasi-real, quasi-ideal entity called Christendom, under the suzerainty of the Pope of Rome.

> It was the church which provided the poor with social services – free food – free hospital treatment. There was for a long while, no other source of education (11:12).

Religious sisters today are still actively engaged in nursing and many have been part of the development of nursing in Southern Africa. In chapter 6 more will be said of these dedicated women and their effect on our own nursing history.

3.1.3 Feudalism

In the chaos which prevailed following the barbarian invasion, towns shrunk, hunger and disease stalked the land, famine was endemic and no person or status was respected. Courts moved from one place to another as the area was denuded of food.

> Towns and monasteries built thick new walls around them; fortified castles began to be built . . . Peasants began to cluster within their protective shadows (11:20).

All this disorder led to the emergence of feudalism in the eighth and ninth centuries CE. In return for some measure of protection from marauding bands, the lord or baron demanded service and taxes from his serfs. In their turn lords owed allegiance to the 'kings' of their areas.

Due to the organisation of social life around the castle of the feudal lord and the position of the lord's wife (who was in charge of the household), it was she who organised what care there was for the sick and also for the wounded, for there was constant warfare during this period of history.

It is difficult for those living today to realise how cut off from each other people were in those times, living their lives in very small social communities. What trade there was was limited, trade routes were dangerous and men had to make do with what they could grow themselves. Weaving was done at home, wool was spun from the wool sheared from sheep. No supermarkets! No refrigerators! No bread to buy from the corner shop! Nursing was still largely based at home and was not organised in the manner in which we understand it today. Travel was limited, but hospices for the care of the weary or sick travellers started growing, attached to monasteries which later became hospitals.

3.1.4 Crusades

The mild rule of the first Muslim conquerors allowed Christian pilgrims to come and go quite freely, but in 1010 CE this state of affairs changed and numerous wars or 'crusades' were mounted. These were thus originally aimed at ensuring the safety of pilgrims visiting the Holy Sepulchre and to set up Christian rule in Palestine. Later on the intent of such *Wars of the Cross* (French *croisade*) changed to religious wars carried on by the nations of Europe against Islam. They actually continued for over two centuries, even though many proved disastrous (32:1586-1587).

The health implications of this movement of people are obvious. The armies of the Crusaders had many killed and wounded in battle. Travel was extremely hazardous and nutrition was poor as food was difficult to carry, obtain or preserve. Epidemic diseases were introduced from East to West. Immunity to newly encountered diseases was low, and since little was known about sanitation, diseases associated with crowded army camp conditions, such as dysentery, were rife.

St Helena (see 2.3.1) and St Paula (see 2.3.5) have already been mentioned as founders of hospitals which cared for pilgrims to the Holy Land.

The military nursing orders had their origin in the early Middle Ages – the Knights Hospitallers of St John of Jerusalem was for instance founded in 1070. Their influence spread in the later Middle Ages (1300-1500 CE), mainly due to the Crusades. The main concern of the military nursing orders was the lives of the Crusaders and not of the poor. Because of their military nature, there were no female members.

☐ *The Knights Hospitallers of St John of Jerusalem.* After the fall of Jerusalem to the Muslims in 1200, the order transferred to Limasol and later to Rhodes in 1310. They settled in Malta in 1530 after being driven away by the Turks again in 1522. The order built hospitals, hospices and hostels. As early as 1617 a board was placed at the head of each bed, on which the doctors' *orders* were written. It is probable that the 'knights' were mainly administrators, and that the actual nursing was done by sergeants.

An order of nursing sisters, the *Sisters of the Knights Hospitallers of St John*, was established at Amalfi in 1050 to care for the female sick and was eventually also re-established at Malta. The Knights Hospitallers of St John brought fresh water to the hospitals of Malta, imposed quarantine and isolation, and had planned methods for the disposal of garbage (1:91).

The headquarters of the order is now in Rome. Many modern orders of St John of Jerusalem still exist and in South Africa it is a secular and philanthrophic organisation with female as well as male members. It owed its founding to the original Knights Hospitallers and part of its work is embodied in the work by the St Johns Ambulance brigade, which is concerned with nursing (especially home nursing), emergency work in accident and other disaster conditions, as well as hospital work. The members of this group are a well-known sight at sportfields, rendering first aid to the injured and indisposed. The badge of the order is still the Maltese cross, white on a black background. The order of sisters, wearing the habit of the Hospitallers, still cares for the sick of Malta.

☐ *The Teutonic Knights* was another order, founded by German merchants in Bremen and Lübeck to alleviate the sufferings of the troops attacking Acre (Palestine) in 1190. A hospital was established and the order of Teutonic Knights of the Hospital of St Mary of Jerusalem was founded. Their mantle was white with a black cross. The members were obliged to tend the sick, protect the poor and wage war against the heathen. The order was secularised in 1525 and eventually suppressed by Napoleon in 1809.

☐ *The Knights of St Lazarus*, one of the oldest of the knightly orders, devoted themselves to the care of lepers. The order was suppressed in 1490. In an attempt at revival they united with the order of *Our Lady of Carmel* and with the *Knights of St Maurice*. There was a female branch, the *Sisters of St Lazarus*, which was later known in France as the 'Dames de St Lazaire'. The French Revolution brought an end to male and female orders in 1772. Very little record exists of the work done by the later revivals (36:5).

3.1.5 Medieval hospitals

Besides the hospitals attached to monasteries, others were built for the care of the sick. The most famous of these were the following:

☐ *Hôtel Dieu* (God's House) founded in Paris in 650 CE, was served by the order of Augustinian sisters, one of the oldest sisterhoods which was formed for nursing only. The routine of washing patients, making beds, giving assistance to patients when needed, feeding and cleaning fell to the lot of the nursing sisters. They were responsible for the kitchens and did all the laundry on the banks of the River Seine, which flows through Paris. Patients were naked in their beds, and the beds held more than one patient (36:6). Apart from the usual day nurses, night nurses were used whose function was more of a 'guarding' nature, namely to protect patients (often from each other). Florence Nightingale was later to visit this hospital when she first started developing an interest in nursing.

☐ *Santo Spirito* Hospital in Rome was founded as early as 717 CE. It was a very large hospital built by order of the Pope to care for the sick.

☐ *St Bartholomew's* Hospital, founded in London in 1123 CE by a Norman monk, was the first hospital in England to receive a Royal Charter. The nursing was provided by Augustinian sisters. The hospital is still in existence, and has become a well-known school of nursing.

☐ *St Thomas'* Hospital, London, had its origins in the priory of St Mary Overie (St Mary the Virgin). An infirmary was attached to the hospital, which was situated on the banks of the Thames at the southern entry to the City of London. It was destroyed by fire but rebuilt in 1106 and renamed and dedicated to St Thomas the Martyr, whence it received its present name. The hospital was eventually separated from the priory (36:7). The hospital was most famous for the nursing school established there by Florence Nightingale in 1860.

☐ *Bethlehem* Hospital, London (Bedlam), originally founded in 1247 by Simon Fitzmary as a priory at Bishopsgate under the ancient St Mary's in Bethlehem, was established by the Knights Hospitallers in 500 CE. The brethren of the priory of St Mary of Bethlehem in Bishopsgate, London, originally cared for about 20 patients. In 1340, however, it was taken over by the mayor and the corporation of the City of London and used as an asylum for the insane. It was later transferred from Bishopsgate, and eventually moved to Kent.

The word *bedlam* has attained connotations of any scene of uproar; it derives from the days when the mentally ill were subject to ravings because of the lack of sophisticated treatment. General scenes of noisy disorder were the order of the day in such places. The patients were not treated very kindly, and were often beaten to try to keep them quiet. After the hospital came under the control of the mayor and corporation there were no doctors and nurses, only keepers (36:7; 32:566).

☐ *Santa Maria Nuova* Hospital, founded in Florence in 1287, was another well-known hospital of the time.

Midwifery in medieval times was entirely in the hands of women. Domestic or 'home' nursing, as well as hospital nursing, was also carried out and it was customary for girls in the upper classes to receive instruction in such knowledge of medical care as was available at the time. This included especially the care of wounds, as they often had to nurse wounded knights.

Country women also learnt about matters such as the use of medicinal herbs, as well as the skills necessary for caring for the sick (36:6).

3.1.6 The School of Salerno

Another feature of the early Middle Ages was the establishment of medical teaching at universities such as Bologna, Montpellier, Naples, Salamanca, Cambridge, Padua and Pisa, the most famous of which was the School of Salerno.

The origin of this medical school is not very clear, although Salerno was known as a health resort from very early times. In 194 CE when it was already famous for the salutary effect of its air and waters, it was annexed to Rome (32:118). It became a famous medical school during the Middle Ages and Frederick of Prussia granted the school the right to license doctors to practise in 1240. It became the place where advice on medicine to laymen of the time was fostered. The writings of the Salerno School were in verse, which could easily be remembered. Practical medical knowledge was thus popularised with straightforward advice that spread throughout the then known world.

Trotula, probably a midwife and the wife of a doctor, is credited with writing a treatise on obstetrics containing advice on what to do before, during and after childbirth, on the treatment of prolapse and polyp of the womb, on the choice of a wet nurse and her diet. Excessive use of salt, garlic, onion and pepper in food were strictly prohibited. This Salerno character found popularity in early English literature as 'Dame Trot' (32:121).

3.1.7 Secular nursing orders

Secular orders were founded to accommodate workers who wished to serve God, without being bound by vows to a monastic life. They could terminate their vows at any time and even return to them later if their circumstances, such as marital status, changed.

☐ *The Order of St Antonines* or *Hospital Brothers of St Anthony* was founded in about 1095. The group consisted of laymen who specialised in caring for patients suffering from St Anthony's fire, which was probably erysipelas. They practised isolation of patients to limit the spread of the disease.

☐ *The Béguines*, a Roman Catholic order of lay sisters, was founded in 1184. They took simple vows and lived in houses called *Béguinages*, but were free to marry or to leave at any time. A hospital adjoined each institution and the lay sisters devoted themselves to nursing, tending the aged and also to educating children. Their most famous houses were at Bruges and Ghent. They also served those who were afflicted as a result of war, famine and epidemics and often converted their homes into hospitals. They worked as volunteer nurses, receiving no payment for their care of the sick. Most of their work was institution oriented, but some of them also served in the community as visiting nurses (32:572; 8:103).

3.1.8 People in the early Middle Ages who had relevance to nursing and nurses

While there were many such people, only the most famous will be mentioned.

☐ *Francis of Assisi* (1182-1226). After a misspent youth, Francis of Assisi founded the mendicant order of Franciscans (mendicant relates to begging; therefore those who possessed nothing of their own and begged in order to support themselves and their work among the poor and needy). The Franciscan Order attracted many followers. Francis preached poverty, chastity and obedience, and devoted himself to prayer and the care of the poor. He also worked among the lepers at Gubbio.

An offshoot of the original order was the Second Franciscan Order (*Poor Clares*, a female order) and the Third Franciscan Order (*Tertiaries*) which is a secular branch consisting of lay people who live in the world, but according to the teachings of St Francis (32:2241).

☐ *Clare* (1194-1253) was the daughter of a rich and noble family of Assisi, and a contemporary of Francis and much influenced by him. She became a nun and eventually settled in Assisi where she founded the Second Franciscan Order, known in England as the *Poor Clares* and in France as *Clarisses* (32:1313). The sisters were not expected to beg themselves, but were supported by donations from the community and by the sale of their products.

☐ *Dominic* (1170-1221) founded the *Order of Preachers* or *Dominicans* at Toulouse in 1215. This was a male order, but prior to this he founded a convent of women in 1207 at Prouille. Dominican sisters of the order have since been very active in the nursing world as well as in other fields of endeavour, such as teaching and pastoral and mission work. A third Dominican order, or the Tertiary Order of lay workers, also came into being (32:1765).

☐ *Anthony of Padua* (1195-1231). He was a disciple of Francis of Assisi and a member of the Franciscan Order (32:252).

☐ *Elizabeth of Hungary* (1207-1231). Elizabeth, a Christian, was the daughter of a king. Her husband was converted when a basket of bread, which Elizabeth was bringing to the poor, turned into red roses when he commanded her to display the contents of her basket. This phenomenon was much celebrated. After the death of her husband she lived as a Franciscan tertiary at Marburg until her death.

3.2 Late Middle Ages (1300-1500CE)

This period, just before the Renaissance or 'Revival of Knowledge', was characterised not only by chaos and confusion in the known world, but also by numerous epidemics. Life was short and hard. Many of the institutions discussed in the previous section still continued into this period and as has been mentioned, some of them still exist today.

The walled castles, which were the refuge for many people against the marauding barbarian tribesmen, became over-populated; people migrated from the land and settled in the growing towns, finding other work to do. A middle class of people gradually emerged. There were shopkeepers, bankers and tradesmen of various types. Some of them became wealthy and powerful, but the lower classes still lived in poverty. Some people became skilled in various crafts which were in demand among the people of these towns. The emergence of craftsmen led to the formation of *guilds*, where people were apprenticed to master craftsmen to learn their skills. A master craftsman had to pass an examination before he could claim this rank. Men following the same craft joined together to form a guild or 'professional body' to help promote high standards and served as a type of labour organisation to fix general conditions of work wages and acceptable standards of work. This type of 'craft' organisation was probably the origin of the apprenticeship system of training for nurses, a system from which the nursing profession is only today emerging into a true professional organisation.

Unfortunately this system of social organisation made little provision for sanitation in these towns and water was often contaminated, and good food was difficult to obtain. This led to the development of slums, which inevitably brought disease.

The various epidemics had a profound influence on the development of care for the sick, and the most important will therefore be discussed in more detail.

3.2.1 The Black Death

This was the name given to pandemics of plague, the worst of which occurred in Europe in 1347-1349, although there were other outbreaks in 1361-1362 and 1369. The Black Death was probably a form of oriental plague which entered

Europe from the East via the ports of Genoa, Venice and Messina.

The Black Death was the worst disaster in the history of the human race, bringing about proportionally more deaths than any World War to date.

The name *Black Death* probably derives from the black spots and buboes on thighs and arms, as well as from the pulmonary form with its bloody, purulent sputum. It was spread by rats and their fleas which infested ships from the East, where plague was endemic.

It brought despair to the people of the time as there was no known cure and the mortality rate was extremely high. It is estimated that the plague of 1347-1349 caused the death of some 25 million people, at least a quarter of the population of the time. It is further estimated that about one third of the population of England perished and it is known that epidemic plague persisted there for 300 years. Family members deserted one another, fleeing in fear. Men deserted their wives, mothers deserted their children, and anyone suspected of being infected was left to die. In certain areas some attempts were made to isolate sufferers and a 40-day period of isolation, from which the word *quarantine* is derived, was introduced in what is now Dubrovnik in 1377. However, as plague was on the whole regarded as a visitation of demons and a punishment for sins, men were resigned to their fate, and in despair did not think any preventative measures would be effective. Margotta (22:142) wrote:

> [A]s the imagined aides of the devil, who was assumed to be the cause of the plague, Jews and lepers became scapegoats, and in many parts were massacred.

The garb of the doctors attending patients included a birdlike mask and long protective clothing (22:141-142).

A description of what could happen in an outbreak of plague is given in Shakespeare's *Romeo and Juliet*, where Romeo is prevented by a plague scare from receiving the message from Friar Lawrence regarding Juliet's induced coma, and so thinks she is actually dead, with tragic consequences.

It is estimated that plague, which started in Asia and Africa, killed about 60 million people in all, which is about a quarter of the total population of the earth. Medical knowledge of the time was unable to cope with it, although physicians of the time were skilled in many ways such as the removing of teeth, setting bones and other forms of treatment (18:287).

Plague presented itself in many forms, especially as huge abscesses in the axillae and groins (bubonic plague), or by coughing up blood in the pneumonic form. The most deadly, namely the septicaemic form, had different symptoms. Many remedies were tried including bleeding, purgatives and enemas in an attempt to rid the body of the 'poison' which must have weakened the sufferers considerably. The buboes were incised, and dressed or covered with hot plasters, but it was soon realised that no treatment was effective and prayer was all that was left.

It is significant that drastic measures were taken, for example in Milan, where the archbishop ordered that the first three houses where plague appeared must be walled up with the dead, sick and healthy inside. This terrible order was carried out and as a result Milan was spared, no further infection passing this barrier (18:285).

Normal life was completely disrupted by the plague. People fled from the cities to isolated areas, farming of land was neglected and animals were not cared for. It goes without saying that this was a terrible period of history.

Faced as we are today with the spread of the (as yet) incurable AIDS (Acquired Immune Deficiency Syndrome) modern medicine knows how the disease is spread, what can be done to prevent infection, how to nurse the patients without the personnel becoming infected, while educating the population in general in all aspects of the disease. Constant high-powered research is being carried out to find a cure for the disease and for a vaccine to prevent its occurrence. This gives people a feeling of some hope.

It is difficult for modern society to imagine what the effects of a terrible epidemic such as the plague may have had on an ignorant 'medical corps' and attendants on the sick who were powerless to help. Modern communications make it possible to know when cases of a dreaded disease appear almost as soon as this happens. Trying to put oneself in the place of the people of those times and think as they did is well-nigh impossible.

3.2.2 Leprosy

This ancient disease was probably brought to Europe by the Crusaders. Leprosy was a generic name given to all manner of skin conditions from scabies and psoriasis to skin cancer as well as to leprosy proper. Despite the fact that some of these conditions were not contagious, all persons labelled as lepers were nevertheless cast out of society and declared dead. The last rites were said and they were isolated or banished to roam away from the rest of the community. They had to give warning of their presence by the ringing of bells and calling 'unclean'. In some cases they were confined in special leprosaria of which there were at one time 19 000 in the Christian world (1:11).

The term lazaretto or lazar house has also been applied to hospitals for lepers, named as such after St Lazarus, the patron saint of lepers, after whom the military order of the Knights of St Lazarus, founded during the crusades, was named (see 3.1.4). It must not be forgotten that many Christians looked on it as their duty to care for lepers, and thus some sufferers received nursing and consolation in their need, despite the generally harsh and cruel attitudes of the times and the fear lepers invoked. These Christian people were caring for those with a terrible need.

Thus human beings were caring for other people, human beings despite the hard, brutal times in which men lived during this time, when pestilence and famine stalked the world.

Although this text places emphasis on the Western world, one should not forget that human beings were being born, living and dying wherever there were people on the earth, often unknown to each other, and separated by high mountains and vast oceans. Care of the young, the sick and wounded was thus not a prerogative of the Western world, and the total picture of health care of various types and in various parts of the world must never be forgotten.

3.2.3 Ergotism – Holy or St Anthony's fire

A strange condition, now known to be caused by a fungus affecting rye, was prevalent from about 1050 to 1129 CE. It caused progressive gangrene of the limbs, ending in severe mutilation and death. It was eventually realised that epidemics only occurred in years when the rye did not ripen properly (22:142).

3.2.4 English sweating sickness (Sudor anglicanus)

This epidemic first broke out in England in 1485 among the troops after the Battle of Bosworth, the last battle between the Houses of Lancaster and York. There were subsequent outbreaks in 1508, 1517, 1528 and 1551. It spread to Calais and occurred in Germany in 1529, and reached as far as Vienna. An outbreak also took place in France in 1718, and another somewhat later.

The onset of the disease was sudden, with malaise and headache, hyperpyrexia, shivering, pain in hands and feet, abdominal pain, delirium, coma and often death. As the name suggests, it was accompanied by profuse perspiration (32:5170). This was probably a form of influenza.

Again, treatment was primitive and probably did more harm than good. Ignorance of the physiology of the body and how to aid the body to help itself probably caused unnecessary deaths. It is interesting to remember that as late as the 1940s it was standard treatment to 'heat' patients suffering from shock, because they felt cold. The fact that fluid loss was caused through sweating, which by warming them increased fluid loss and the shocked state, was not recognised until later. The author remembers the placing of metal cradles with electric light bulbs inside over patients suffering from shock, as standard treatment! Nowadays one only prevents further heat loss, and replaces lost fluid because of better understanding of the physiology involved in shock.

3.2.5 Syphilis

A serious epidemic of syphilis broke out in Naples in 1495 and from there spread throughout Europe (1:12). Baly suggests that a new strain of spirochaete came from an unknown source, probably even from the 'New World' (Americas). Whatever the cause, there was an upsurge in Europe which caused untold misery.

3.3 Conclusion

In conclusion, the despair that prevailed in this period of history gave rise to several strange patterns of social behaviour such as the *dancing mania*, a hysterical manifestation which broke out in Germany after the plague spread through the Low Countries and northern France; as well as the appearance of the *Flagellants*, who wore dark cloaks with scarlet crosses on their breasts. They were fanatics who went about in bands, flogging themselves in the belief that the Lord would be moved to compassion by their self-inflicted suffering, and stop the advance of the plague or at least spare them. The Flagellants also founded hospitals at Bologna, Imola, Ferrara and Treviso (32:141).

The famous Passion Play of Oberammergau in Bavaria owes its origin to a vow made by the inhabitants that if they were spared from the plague, they and their descendants would celebrate God's mercy by producing a passion play once a decade.

Another strange social phenomenon was the heavy drinking and debauchery in Florence during a plague epidemic, presumably in the belief that as life would be short, it might as well be merry.

Other infectious diseases which were rife during these times were typhus, smallpox, tuberculosis and gonorrhoea. There was also a great deal of malnutrition, including avitaminosis, scurvy and rickets.

Typhus decimated armies and was prevalent among troops, in prisons, hospitals and asylums. If the misery of wars, famine, poor sanitation and overcrowding is added to this, it seems a wonder that the human race survived. To attain the age of 20 years was quite an achievement. The nurse of the late 20th century may have difficulty imagining such conditions, as many of the infectious diseases are well under control nowadays and some have even been eradicated. One should keep in mind that the neglect of immunisation services, sanitation and basic care all result in major health hazards. Poor social conditions usually lead to overcrowding and its attendant health problems, while severe drought or floods cause famine.

Health services are responsible for the health of the population and one step backwards can bring disaster, even in this day and age. Although man has walked on the moon, he must constantly be on the alert for possible health disasters which may destroy the general complacency that all is well on the health front.

In the late Middle Ages (ca 1380) the *Brethren of the Common Life,* a secular order of men, was founded by Gerard Groot. They could leave whenever they liked, but had to keep the vows of chastity, poverty and obedience as long as they remained Brethren. At first they devoted themselves to the care of the sick poor, visiting them in their homes, but later branched out into teaching. There were also *Sisters of the Common Life,* who, although they took no vows, devoted themselves to the care of the sick, especially to the care and teaching of sick children (32:816).

The most famous nursing saint of the late Middle Ages was Catherine of Siena (1347-1380), who belonged to the Dominican Order and worked among the poor. She was noted for her care of persons with plague, leprosy and other distressing diseases (8:102). St Catherine is generally regarded as the patron saint of nursing.

By the late Middle Ages medicine, developing along the lines established by the School of Salerno, passed entirely into the hands of laymen. Until the 12th century monks performed surgery with the assistance of visiting barbers. However, a *Lateran Council* later forbade monks to perform surgery as it involved the shedding of human blood. The formation of a Guild of Surgeons was the result (1:13). The Church also frowned on dissection of human bodies, with the result that ignorance of human anatomy still prevailed.

From 1500 CE hospitals thus began to pass from the hands of the Church to the civil authorities. Many well-organised institutions and hospitals were established where it was possible to give devoted care according to the needs of the sick and the knowledge of the times.

Nursing itself was not organised in any noticeable way, but what did exist, apart from the mother-family-neighbourhood type of care, was carried out by various religious nursing orders. Care rather than cure was the dominant feature of the nursing of the day and subsequently there was nothing scientific about it.

4

FROM 1500 TO 1800 CE

4.1 Setting the scene

It is necessary to review the background against which nursing was practised during 1500-1800 CE. Hale (14:11) made the following observations.

> Human nature does not change much. Man has always liked food and warmth, raised families, felt happier when the sun shone than when it rained, wanted peace and fought wars, created delicate works of art and committed violent crimes.

The period which is now under review is certainly no different where the human being is considered. It was, however, a time of significant changes and may perhaps have been the time when *modern man*, as the 20th century regards him, was born.

4.1.1 Historical events of significance

This text does not purport to give a full account of the history of the world, but nursing did not occur nor develop into what it is today in isolation from events which took place at the time. It is for this reason that a short summary of significant historical events of the period is given to afford perspective to nursing developments.

This period followed the Black Death 'epoch', when the death of one quarter to one third of the population of the Western world in about two and a half years left the remaining population reeling. Medicine could not cure, and it was felt by many that the Church had failed the flock in a time of disaster. Medieval man was disillusioned and depressed (1:10) and the time was ripe for the rebirth of learning.

4.1.1.1 The Renaissance

This movement, which started in Italy, was a period during which man started to display an intense curiosity about *man* as such, particularly due to a reawakening of individualism, a new freedom of thought and action, and a new interest in the workings and mysteries of nature and science. A broadening and sharpening of the critical faculty occurred. Art was transformed and new fields were opened up in every branch of science. With all this enquiry medicine gained a true scientific basis (32:4611-4614).

4.1.1.2 The Reformation

The revolution which took place in the Western Church in the 16th century was called the *Reformation*. It was a logical development from the Renaissance which had fostered a critical attitude, through which many practices of the established Church and its doctrine were called into question. Some of the prominent figures in the Reformation were Martin Luther (1483-1546) in Germany, Ulrich Zwingli (1484-1546) in Switzerland, Jean Calvin (1509-1564) in France and Switzerland and John Knox (1513-1572) in Scotland.

The effect of the Reformation was to break up the unity of Christendom and the formation of many Protestant churches. It also brought about reform in the Roman Catholic Church itself (32:4595-4597). The dissolution of the monasteries in England by Henry VIII had a considerable effect on those areas where nuns had practised some form of organised nursing in convent hospitals and led to a decline in the care of the sick and the so-called 'Dark Age of Nursing'.

4.1.1.3 Exploration

Hale (14(b):11) says the following about the Renaissance: 'The Renaissance voyages of discovery rank as one of history's two or three most important phenomena in terms of their effect on the modern world'.

Looking for unknown lands beyond Europe increased knowledge of the planet and corrected many wrong ideas of the times.

> Discovery led to colonisation and settlement . . . new wealth, new products, new opportunities, new problems, new ways of thinking, new commitments, and to the creation of new nations (14(b):11).

Exploration did not really lead to the 'discovery' of barren lands. Many had thriving populations, established civilisations, some even possessed books and maps describing their countries, and 'this information was gratefully taken over by the European voyagers' (14(b):11). It did lead to a new conception of the previous erroneous beliefs of the world, due to the 'discovery' of 'new' worlds and eventually the circumnavigation of the globe.

Leadership in exploration was taken almost exclusively by Portugal, Spain, England, France and the Netherlands. Well-known people in the history of exploration were Bartolomeu Dias, who rounded the Cape of Storms in 1488, later known as the Cape of Good Hope, and actually landed in Algoa Bay. Vasco da Gama (1469-1524) reached India in 1498, having rounded the Cape in 1497. Christopher Columbus (1451-1506) made four voyages west, discovering Cuba, Haiti (Hispaniola) and Dominica, eventually reaching the mainland of South America in 1498. On his last voyage he explored the Gulf of Mexico in 1502. These lands were colonised by Spain. Ferdinand Magellan (1480-1521) was a Portuguese navigator who discovered the strait bearing his name in 1520, and was the first European to navigate in the Pacific Ocean. Although he was killed in the Philippines, one of his ships returned to Spain, thus being the first ship to circumnavigate the globe.

Other important explorers of this period include Amerigo Vespucci (1451-1512) who made several voyages to the New World between 1497 and 1504, exploring the coast of South America as far as the River Plate and realised that America was a new continent and not the Indies as was at first thought.

Martin Frobisher (1535-1594), an Englishman, made several voyages of discovery first on the northern shores of Africa and then the northern part of the American continent, searching for a north-west passage to the East. Francis Drake (1545-1596) made several voyages to the West Indies and circumnavigated the globe from 1577 to 1581. He played a leading part in the defeat of the Spanish Armada, and died of dysentery on a voyage to the West Indies. Hale (14(b):19) touches on an important aspect of the voyages of discovery in the following quotation.

> Outsailing, outshooting and outwitting peoples who had no wish to be explored, let alone exploited, the Europeans thrust their way across the world, nowhere encountering either equal technological ability or an ideology that would support effective resistance.

Much of the exploration was motivated by a search for gold and spices and the desire to spread Christianity. The ships were small, life aboard was brutal, food was atrocious and sailors were payed a few pennies a day (Hale, 14(a):93). Health suffered and some of the settlements, which eventually led to colonisation such as at the Cape of Good Hope in 1652, actually came into being because of the need to establish a place where fresh food and water could be obtained and sick crewmen could be left to be 'nursed' back to health where possible. Scurvy was the scourge of those voyaging long distances, because of the absence of fresh fruit and vegetables. Thus the European settlement at the Cape was established due to an occupational health hazard.

4.1.1.4 Colonisation

The Spaniards who explored and conquered Peru and Mexico, under leaders such as Francisco Pizarro (1475-1541) and Hernán Cortes (1485-1547), suffered many hardships. Journeys into the interior were hazardous. Food was very scarce, climatic conditions varied from frozen highlands with icy winds to the hot and humid tropics, and soldiers and others accompanying the explorers and conquerors, fell ill and died as did local 'Indians', so called because of the belief of early explorers that the continent of America was in fact India. The latter were pressed into service as porters and herders of pigs and other livestock, which were taken on the expeditions in the hope that they would provide food.

The Portuguese cultivated sugar plantations in Brazil, and imported Negro slaves from Africa to work them. Thus extensive slavery was one of the evils brought about by exploration and subsequent colonisation.

The British, French and Dutch colonised the northern part of the American continent, New Guinea, Australia and New Zealand. James Cook (1728-1779) was the first explorer to take possession of areas in Australasia, which had originally been discovered by the Dutch.

Because of the differing interests of nations, colonial wars were fought frequently, as well as wars with the indigenous populations of the discovered lands.

The Cape was originally settled by the Dutch, although it changed hands a few times during the course of history, while India was conquered and colonised by the French, British and Portuguese, as were parts of the Central African continent.

Missionaries played a large part in colonisation, taking the word of God to outlying places. After the Reformation many missionaries were Protestants, and not specifically members of the Catholic Church, as was the case in the first Christianising expeditions. The Reformation also caused people to settle in distant lands to escape religious persecution, in addition to poor social conditions. In taking the word of God to far-away places, they often established mission hospitals to care for the sick who came to them for help. These hospitals often consisted of one primitive hut, but expanded to provide extensive health services after a period of time.

Colonisation was not aimed at bringing 'civilisation' to so-called primitive people, but was in fact mostly inspired by commercial interests. Except in areas such as the Cape where the establishment of a hospital was one of the duties of the Dutch East India Company responsible for the first White settlement, health care was only incidental. Even the Cape settlement was commercially inspired, as the loss of life in crew-members (due to ill health) endangered the safety of the ships and caused financial loss to the Company.

The health of the indigenous colonised people was often adversely affected by the people from distant lands as they brought diseases such as measles, diphtheria and scarlet fever with them, to which the native inhabitants had never been exposed. The diseases decimated populations because of their lack of resistance to the 'imported' infections. Children of colonists, too, were often badly affected by such diseases, as they had previously been isolated and thus had no chance to build up a herd immunity. It must be remembered that ships had no health laws to which they had to adhere and no real quarantine of epidemic diseases was known.

4.1.1.5 The French Revolution

The French Revolution which propagated the philosophy of liberty, equality and fraternity, started in 1789 and was accompanied by much bloodshed. The absolute power of the monarchy was overthrown. Louis XVI and his wife Marie Antoinette were executed, as were many other aristocrats in addition to some of the prominent revolutionary leaders and others. A republican form of government was established, though interrupted for a while when Napoleon Bonaparte made himself emperor of France. Wars were constantly being waged, with all the attendant human misery including starvation, wounds, maiming, dysentery, typhus and other diseases. Many people fled the country.

4.1.1.6 Colonial America

The first British colony was settled in 1586 in Virginia by Sir Walter Raleigh. The explorers returning to Europe from the first ill-fated settlement brought back tobacco. Thus, the origins of the present health hazard, smoking, have deep roots in history. People fleeing from religious persecution formed settlements in 1620 in New England, and the Quakers under William Penn settled in what is today known as Pennsylvania.

Canada was first settled by the French and conquered in 1759 by the British. Such forceful occupations, and war against the Indians and the American War of Independence from 1774 to 1783, in which Britain was defeated, also brought its attendant miseries to the New World. The latter war eventually led to the formation of the United States of America. Canada, however, remained British.

Native medicines brought to Europe from the Americas, as a result of exploration and colonisation included quinine, cascara sagrada and balsam from Peru. The first European hospital on the American continent, the Hospital of the Immaculate Conception, was established by Cortes in 1524.

French religious nursing sisters (Augustinians) established the Hôtel Dieu, the first of its kind, in Quebec in 1639 (8:143). A hospital of some sort was established in the British Colony of Virginia in 1620 (1:145), while the first hospital in 'New Netherlands' (today's New York) was established on Manhattan Island in 1658. This was the beginning of New York's Bellevue Hospital (8:147).

The first hospital on the southern African continent appears to have been erected in Mozambique in March 1508 (27(a):10), where slaves attended to the needs of the sick. In 1682 a new hospital, run by the Nursing Brothers of the Order of St John of God, replaced the original one.

The Dutch East India Company appointed many surgeons and even a few physicians to their ships, while the first temporary tent hospital was established at the Cape of Good Hope in 1652 (27(a):ch 3).

During the time of the Renaissance in Europe, the Aztec civilisation (destroyed by the Spaniard Hernán Cortes in 1521) and the Ming dynasty in China rose and flourished.

4.1.2 Significant social changes

The establishment of the movable printing press by Gutenberg in the mid 15th century, made it possible for knowledge to reach many more people of all social classes. This led to an upsurge in learning and scientific knowledge especially, with people acquiring a wide variety of new skills.

A new middle class came into being, which was completely different from medieval feudalism. Businessmen, banks and exchanges all had their origin in this period.

The purpose of education changed in the belief that children should be educated to become men equipped to fit knowledgeably into all walks of life (14(a):55). Education was almost exclusively geared to males, and women (with few exceptions) were expected to bring up their children and run their homes with the result that few women acquired an education (14(a):58).

It must be borne in mind that the changes took place very gradually and imperceptibly. Human life was still cheap and torture, burning of witches at the stake, and barbarous death penalties were practised for what seem to be quite trivial offences according to modern norms. Cities grew and nations began to emerge as coherent entities, sometimes in the form of small states, which were later to become amalgamated into the type of nation we know today.

The Industrial Revolution was brought about by the remarkable and rapid development of industrial technology. Weaving and spinning which had been cottage industries before the invention of the *flying shuttle* in 1733 and the *spinning jenny* in 1764, now came to be mass produced. This led to the establishment of factories and the virtual elimination of cottage industries. Together with the exploitation of the coal-mines, this was responsible for tremendous social change due to the congregation of masses of people around mills and coal-mines, often in poor housing conditions. Many of the factories exploited the workers, who worked long hours in poor conditions. Child labour was a common phenomenon. These conditions combined to bring poor health and misery to many, compounded by the fact that no occupational medicine was practised, nor was there any knowledge of health hazards in manufacturing processes.

Although it was the practice of ancient nations to enslave prisoners of war and others, it was only with the discovery of America and its colonisation that another form of slavery arose, when 'Christian' nations purchased African Negroes for employment in the mines and plantations of the New World.

The captured slaves were brought to the New World, where the survivors were sold, in slave ships in appalling conditions. Slave trading was eventually outlawed in the early 19th century, but internal slave trade continued to flourish in the United States of America for some time (32:4981). The abolition of slavery in America will be discussed in the next chapter under the heading 'The American Civil War'.

4.1.3 Important scientific and medical advances

Because writing and printing made the recording of events and the dissemination of knowledge possible, there is a wealth of information available from this period. A summary of important changes in medicine and science and a brief mention of some of the people who left their mark on the development of modern medicine, with an indication of their specific contribution, follow.

4.1.3.1 Lenses and microscopes

It is now agreed that the first microscope was invented by Johannes and Zacharias Jansen of Middelburg in Holland in 1590. Antoni van Leeuwenhoek (1612-1723) of Delft modified and improved the microscope, grinding his own lenses. Because of the time he spent observing water, small insects and tissue through the microscope, he initiated the science of microbiology in 1676 by describing the microscopic animals which he observed in these substances (22:212).

4.1.3.2 Blood transfusions

The purpose of transferring blood from the donor to a recipient was known in England and France in the 17th century (32:680). The first authentically recorded blood transfusion on human beings was performed in June 1667, when nine ounces of blood from a lamb was given to a teenage boy (8:124). Attempts to transfuse blood from one human being to another were made in the early 19th century in England and Germany, often with disastrous results (32:680).

4.1.3.3 Obstetric forceps

A family of Huguenot immigrants to England, the Chamberlens, developed and used the first known *obstetric forceps*.

Peter Chamberlen I, the second generation of this family (his father William had fled to England with his family in 1569) was physician to James the First of England and his wife Anne, and invented the obstetric forceps. This instrument remained a closely guarded secret of the family until the last of the Chamberlens, Hugh, died in 1728. Other members of this family, Peter Chamberlen II, a brother of Peter Chamberlen I, Peter Chamberlen III, a son of Peter II who succeeded his uncle as court physician and delivered Charles II in 1630 and Hugh Chamberlen, the eldest son of Peter III, all figured prominently in midwifery and obstetric practice. Peter Chamberlen III attempted to organise female midwives into a company with himself as president. Hugh Chamberlen attended Queen Mary, the wife of James II at the birth of the Old Pretender and of Princess (later Queen) Anne.

The 'secret instrument' of the Chamberlens was used by them for many years and enabled them to deal with difficult deliveries more effectively than anyone had before them. They remained hidden after Hugh Chamberlen's death in 1700 until 1813 when they were discovered, and are now in possession of the Royal College of Obstetricians and Gynaecologists. Richard Manningham who was one of the first to introduce lying-in wards to hospitals in England in 1739, and Sir Fielding Ould, who helped to found the Dublin School for Midwifery in 1710, William Giffard (1726) and Edmund Chapman (1733) began to specialise in the subject and to develop the practice of midwifery or obstetrics as a pursuit for men (32:164).

4.1.3.4 Instruments for measuring body temperature

Santorio Santorio (1561-1636), a physician who studied at Padua, was regarded as the founder of physiology of metabolism, introducing into physiology exact methods of measurement, pulse counting, temperature determination and weighing. In his writing (1626) he records the first use of the thermometer in the study of disease (32:4802). The thermometers in use had been devised by members of the Academia del Cimento and by Santorio. The modern clinical thermometer only dates from the latter half of the 19th century (22:217).

4.1.3.5 Vaccination

Although inoculation against smallpox was known in China and also in Europe in the 11th century, it was Edward Jenner (1749-1823), who worked as a country doctor for many years, who actually realised vaccination against smallpox. He observed that milkmaids who had had cowpox did not get smallpox, which claimed about 600 000 lives annually in Europe in the 18th century. Through careful experimentation Jenner was able to produce immunity to the disease by the use of cowpox vaccine. The publication of his findings in 1796 began a new era in preventive medicine (22:210).

4.1.3.6 The circulation of the blood

Although there had been many theories of how this occurred, it was the Englishman William Harvey, a student at Padua, who was eventually able to give an accurate description of how blood circulated in the human body. Although his discovery dates back to 1616, his findings were not published until 1628. It was Marcello Malpighi (1628-1694) who proved the existence of capillaries in 1661, by using the newly discovered microscope (22:210).

4.1.3.7 Human anatomy

In order to paint and sculpt the human body accurately, Leonardo da Vinci (1452-1519) and other artists dissected human corpses and many drew what they observed at these dissections. Artists bought their paints from apothecaries, which brought them into close contact with physicians. It is thus not surprising that the son of an apothecary, the Fleming Andreas Vesalius, born in Brussels in 1514, seriously questioned the teachings of Galen, who had until then been considered the authority on anatomy. Vesalius's *De humani corporis fabrica libri septem* (Seven books on the structure of the human body) was a milestone in medical history, although it evoked a storm at the time (22:152-165).

4.1.3.8 Other notable persons

Paracelsus (Phillipus Aureolus Theophrastus Bombastius von Hollenheim, 1493-1541) was a Swiss-born medical practitioner of repute who broke with tradition in Basle by lecturing in German instead of the customary Latin. He was responsible for the introduction of new ideas in the Germanic countries, while Ambroise Paré (1517-1590), originally a barber-surgeon, led the emergence of new ideas in France and introduced sensible, rational treatment of wounds. He is also famous for saying 'I treated him, God healed him' (22:178-187). Thomas Sydenham (1624-1689), a British physician, made a great contribution to the field of general medicine. He advocated fresh air in the sickroom and the simplification of medical prescriptions, among other things (8:127).

Giovanni Battista Morgagni (1682-1771), a professor at the University of Padua, is regarded as having been the founder of scientific pathological anatomy (22:231). Gabriel Daniel Fahrenheit (1686-1736), a German physicist, introduced improvements into the thermometer, using mercury instead of alcohol. He devised the Fahrenheit scale of temperature measurement (32:2787). Antoine-Laurent Lavoisier (1743-1794), a victim of the French Revolution, is famous as the father of modern chemistry and as an eminent physiologist who completed the study of the physiology of respiration (22:232,233).

John Hunter (1728-1793) was a Scottish surgeon and anatomist who is regarded as the founder of surgical pathology, while James Lind (1716-1794), a British doctor, became a naval physician and worked for 25 years in that post. He discovered that scurvy could be prevented by the use of lemon juice (hence the nickname of 'Limey' for British seamen), and was responsible for the eradication of scurvy from the British Navy.

4.1.3.9 Guilds

During the 12th century groups of craftsmen organised themselves into *guilds* so as to protect their trading interests in England, Germany and Switzerland. Since Pope Honorius III had forbidden the clergy to practise medicine, this passed to the laity, and physicians also began to organise themselves into professional bodies, with rights that were protected by law in much the same way as guilds did. No one could enter a profession without having completed a special course of study and proving that they had attained the requisite level of knowledge. This improved the status of physicians in society, and was the first step in the organisation of the medical profession (22:146). It was not until the end of the 19th century that nursing was to become organised similarly.

4.2 Nursing during this period

With the dissolution of monasteries in England, Germany and other Protestant countries, nothing was done to found hospitals for the sick, or to establish nursing orders to replace the monks and nuns (19). Thus the provision of good nursing care based on feeling and not on knowledge, once again devolved on the home. This period is known as the Dark Age of Nursing, since hospitals, deprived of religious sisters with no substitute staff, became squalid places of horror, with 'dirty, ugly, unwhole hags as attendants' (8:129).

Hospitals, many of which had been closed, were unsavoury places, dirty with conditions which were the breeding ground for epidemics. Several patients were placed in the same bed, regardless of what was wrong with them. As the religious orders were no longer able to function, the hospital attendants were drawn from the lowest type of women, who were dirty, drunk, uneducated to the point of illiteracy and immoral. Some were actually convicted criminals who were sent to 'nurse' the sick instead of serving their goal sentences (8:193).

Some hospitals were better than others but the situation as a whole was grim.

In *Martin Chuzzlewit*, Charles Dickens introduced the character *Sairey Gamp*, a nurse who attended the sick in their homes, supposedly looking after the 'woman in childbirth or preparing a dead body for burial'. Dickens describes her as a fat, dirty, gin-drinking old hag, smelling of spirits and snuff. According to the author who created her, she was a self-styled midwife, and he depicts her as a typical so-called 'nurse' of the day.

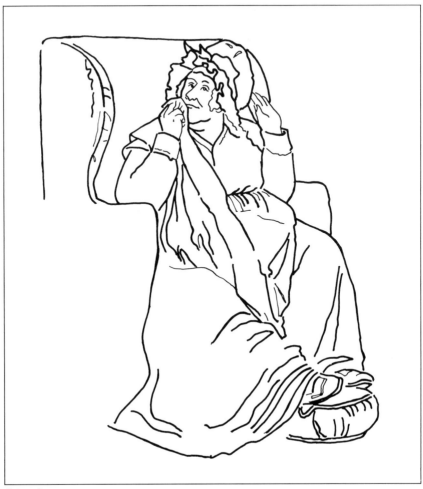

Sairey Gamp

Some of the larger hospitals in England which were taken over by the City of London and run by civilians included St Thomas' Hospital, where Florence Nightingale was to make her mark and St Bartholomew's, both still existing today.

Nursing was at a low ebb, women had no say in hospital management or the management of what 'nursing' there was. This was truly a Dark Age in the history of nursing.

The modern nurse may have difficulties to think herself into the conditions which prevailed at this period, but should, nonetheless, remember that it was the need for the reform of such conditions and poor conditions in society generally that led to the emergence of modern nursing.

In countries where the religious sisterhoods continued to exist, standards of nursing care did not fall so low in the institutions which they controlled.

Lay 'nurses' performed menial tasks; they were rough, cared little for the people for whom they were supposed to be caring; the pay was poor and the working hours were long. No one became a nurse who could possibly make a living in any other way, including prostitution. There was no social status at all.

4.2.1 Prominent figures

Despite the difficult times for nursing there were people who started to evolve new ideas about organisation and control of the care of the sick, which had an effect on later developments in nursing. The following section will mention these people and their achievements briefly.

4.2.1.1 St John of God

Although he was born in Portugal in 1495, he spent most of his life in Spain, first as a shepherd, then a soldier, and then again a shepherd. He eventually founded an order of brothers which became known as the Brothers Hospitallers of St John of God. This order was devoted to the care of the sick, and in particular of sick children and the mentally ill. A hospital was founded in Granada where patients had beds to themselves, a very unusual practice at the time. Those with contagious diseases were isolated, and an out-patient section was started. Brothers of the order went to America as early as 1602 (8:138, 139).

Brothers of this religious order of nursing monks extended their work and built hospitals all over the then civilised world.

4.2.1.2 Francis de Sales (1567-1622)

With the help of Madame de Chantal this French bishop founded an organisation of women who could be regarded as one of the earliest visiting nursing groups. They were not bound by external vows, but were devoted to the care of the sick at home. The order was known as the Order of Visitation of Mary (32:2241; 8:134).

4.2.1.3 Vincent de Paul (1581-1660)

He was a French priest who devoted himself to the relief of the poor, establishing what he called 'confréries de charité' (associations of charity) in various towns in France (32:5336). He established a group of nurses, *Dames de Charité*, who visited the sick poor, attending to their needs. Louise de Marillac (later Madame le Gras) assisted in teaching and supervising this group. Another secular group founded by Vincent de Paul was that for hospital care established at the Hôtel Dieu in Paris, where the sick had been neglected and hygienic standards were poor. Here again he was assisted by Louise de Marillac. This group was the Vincentian Sisters of Charity (Les Filles de Charité) established in 1633 (1:20, 21; 32:5536).

4.2.1.4 Louise de Marillac (Madame le Gras)

She was a contemporary of Vincent de Paul, a well-educated woman who became a pious penitent of Vincent de Paul. She was to become greatly interested in the work among the sick and undertook the administration and supervision of the nursing orders founded by Vincent de Paul. She became the first sister of charity of St Vincent de Paul. This movement to organise care of the sick was the first secular movement after the Reformation which combined the principles of discipline, devotion and training for the practice of nursing (1:21). Madame le Gras was the first supervisor of those nurses who worked in the community, that is, *community nurses*.

4.2.1.5 John Howard (1726-1790)

John Howard was an English Baptist who became famous for his interest in prison reform and especially in prison hygiene. He advocated separation of the sick prisoners from the healthy, bathing and the provision of medical care (1:21, 22).

Many people have been omitted from the list, but the mentioned figures give an idea of what new lines of thought were developing.

4.2.2 General observations

Although this period of history saw the birth of modern medicine with the studies undertaken at the various universities (14a:91), the practice of medicine was not very extensive among the general populace. Probably more people died in hospitals than were cured, because of ignorance of disease causation and elements of community health such as sanitation. Wards were mostly small, overcrowded and poorly ventilated. Hospitals were dirty and the diet of patients was poor and monotonous. Ambulant patients often had to help in caring for the bedridden, and the standard of care was very poor indeed. Puerperal sepsis was rife and infant mortality extremely high.

The care of the insane was limited to protection of the community by incarcerating the insane. Personal treatment was inhumane and often cruel.

Nevertheless the scene was set for the true scientific age of medicine and the emergence of modern nursing, together with a growing concern for the health and welfare of the masses.

Some interest was already being shown in infant welfare, while midwifery remained largely the prerogative of female midwives. The Chamberlens were classified as 'male midwives' and licensed to practise as such.

John Howard was already engaged in humanitarian work, and Elizabeth Fry (1780-1845), who spans this period and the following, was a reformer who had an influence on nursing. Her contribution will be discussed in the following chapter.

In the field of nursing education there were already attempts to bring this into organised existence. In 1630 Vincent de Paul expressed a wish that the religious sisters be *taught nursing*; Professor Franz May of Mannheim, Germany, persuaded some of the authorities responsible for the running of hospitals to provide a series of lectures to successive groups of nursing attendants, and actually gave a series of lectures for nurses at the University of Heidelberg in 1797. In 1793 the Italian professor Sannazara pleaded for more understanding of the fact that the role of the nurse was of great importance in the care of the sick. Dr Valentine Seaman also gave a series of lectures to nurses at a New York hospital in 1798. The real emergence of modern nursing education also took place in the next century and will therefore be discussed in more detail in the next chapter.

5

FROM 1800 ONWARDS – THE EMERGENCE OF MODERN NURSING

A background of the general history of the world is essential if the changes that took place in nursing during this period are to be seen in proper perspective.

5.1 Historical overview

The year 1800 coincided with the beginning of a period of political revolution, alongside the general enlightenment throughout the world. This merged into an age of social revolution, which began about the mid 19th century. However, these periods cannot be categorised into specific epochs without overlaps.

Many of the great philosophers, such as Immanuel Kant, had already brought radical intellectualism into being. As early as 1784 Kant wrote the following in an article: 'Dare to know! Have the courage to use your own intelligence' (12:11). Science 'had broken loose from the moorings of tradition' and a coalition of science and philosophy led the best minds of the age into scientific enquiry and gave science the sanction of reason (12:15).

Many new perspectives were gained, particularly in the natural sciences. Technical skills and artistic endeavour reached new heights.

In 1807 the slave trade was abolished in the British Empire. During this time Britain was involved in the Peninsular War and Europe, too, was in a constant state of war as Napoleon Bonaparte came to power in France in 1799 and his desire to conquer Europe embroiled practically the whole Western world.

Queen Victoria ascended the British throne in 1831, while the independence of the Transvaal was recognised by Britain in 1852. During 1853-1856 Britain and France became involved in the Crimean War against Russia. The American Civil War started in 1861.

Both the Crimean War and the American Civil War were important to medical and nursing history. In the Crimean War troops were badly affected by cholera and Florence Nightingale (see section 5.4.4) made her great contribution to military hospital organisation and hospital hygiene, and to re-establishing nursing as a respected profession. The American Civil War is often regarded as the first 'modern' war because of the large-scale use of modern technology.

The American Civil War (1861-1865) was a long, costly, bloody war (32:5448) in which half a million lives were lost, while tens of thousands of soldiers returned with their health permanently impaired (32:5464). Slavery was eventually abolished in the United States of America as a result of this war.

It was towards the end of the American Civil War that Lister (see section 5.3.5) introduced antiseptic surgery in Glasgow and Mendel's experiments on heredity were conducted (see section 5.3.2). The Salvation Army was also founded in 1878.

Wars continued to trouble the world in the East as well as in Europe and the West. The Red Cross was formed in 1864, an organisation which owes its establishment to the Swiss banker, Jean Henri Dunant. The sufferings of the wounded at the Battle of Solferina in Italy (June 1859) in the war between France and Austria (Rome was, at that time, occupied by France) resulted in his publishing an article 'Un Souvenir de Solferino' in 1862 which urged the formation of permanent voluntary aid societies to succour the wounded in times of war. As a result, an international conference followed by a diplomatic congress in Geneva was held in 1864 and the Red Cross was founded. This organisation went from strength to strength and today offers relief of suffering in any condition of disaster, whether induced by war or not.

The Red Cross is a neutral international organisation, and its emblem is the flag of Switzerland reversed, that is, a red cross against a white background. In some countries where the symbol of a cross is not acceptable, the organisation uses other approved symbols such as the red crescent in Moslem countries and in Iran the red lion and sun.

In 1881 Pasteur's work on anthrax immunisation was undertaken (section 5.3.5). War was still 'endemic' in Europe and on the whole of the African continent. The Anglo-Boer War began in South Africa in 1899, lasting until 1902. The health implications of this war are discussed in chapter 6, which focuses on the history of nursing in South Africa.

The year 1903 saw the first flight of a machine that was heavier than air. The development in the field of aviation in the following eight decades has been nothing short of spectacular. In 1919 the first direct flight across the Atlantic Ocean took place. Travel has become ever more rapid, and has brought with it its own health problems to a 'shrinking' world.

1906 was the year of a terrible earthquake in San Francisco and, at the same time, marked the discovery of vitamins by FG Hopkins.

In 1910 the Union of South Africa was established. Florence Nightingale died the same year. During this period the Panama Canal was completed. This venture had many health hazards and in 1905 work on the canal was eventually taken over by the United States of America. Traffic started passing through in 1914, but it was only officially opened in 1920. Yellow fever and malaria, two health hazards that delayed work considerably, were controlled during this period (32:4158, 4159).

In 1914 the First World War broke out with the Allies of Great Britain and its dominions, France, the Low Countries, and later the United States of America on one side and Germany, Austria, Hungary and Turkey on the other. This war, which ended in 1918, was largely a matter of trench warfare, although gas and aeroplanes were used as means of attacking the enemy.

The year 1917 saw the Russian Revolution, which eventually led to the establishment of the Union of Soviet Socialist Republics.

During the period from 1920 to 1938 there was no real peace in the world. There were various 'smaller' wars, with the ascendancy of Nazism in Germany under Adolf Hitler and Fascism in Italy under Benito Mussolini. The Spanish Civil War was also fought during this time.

The period from 1939 to 1945 covered the Second World War, in which Britain and France, the Low Countries, Greece and Yugoslavia, joined by Russia in June 1941 and the United States of America in December 1941, fought against Germany, Italy, Japan (from 1941) and Turkey.

The first atomic bomb was dropped on Japan in 1944. The end of the war saw the formation of the United Nations Organisation, which organised several health-related activities.

Nuclear power continued to be developed and was also put to peaceful use, not only for the generation of power but, in the medical field, for the treatment of diseases.

During the next four decades the following events of importance occurred:

The *Korean War* (1950-1953) was a struggle between communist and anti-communist forces. The ideology of communism, however, continued to spread.

Despite the general belief that man was not capable of breaking the record for running the mile in four minutes, Roger Bannister's record has been bettered several times since 1954, when he first broke the four minute barrier.

The war in *Vietnam* took place, America becoming involved in 1960. This war, which lasted until 1973, caused a great deal of suffering and came to an inconclusive end.

It was during this time that the *colonies* of the *British Empire* gradually *received independent status*, some breaking all bonds with the British Commonwealth to become republics outside the Commonwealth. Other colonial powers also granted independence to their former territories.

Space exploration proceeded apace, with the first man walking on the moon on 21 July 1969. Satellites became commonplace and were used for sophisticated communication systems.

Student unrest in Europe and America was a feature of the seventies, while *Northern Ireland*, particularly Belfast and Londonderry, saw increased disturbances from 1969 onwards. This conflict and the consequent deaths and misery still persist.

Israel eventually emerged as an independent Jewish state in 1948, becoming involved in conflict with Egypt and more recently with the Lebanon. Its existence has been the source of constant dispute and attack by the Arab states. Wars have certainly not been banished from the earth!

The Shah of Iran was deposed and *Iran* became a Republic accompanied by much unrest and bloodshed. War has broken out between Iran and Iraq.

The whole period was full of so much change and so many events of significance that it is extremely difficult to attempt a coherent summary. There have been such advances in technology and such devastating developments in the means of destruction that man can use against his fellow human beings, that it is almost impossible to assimilate and to recognise the implications of all the changes that have occurred.

The planet earth has never been free from conflict at some point or other, with weaponry so sophisticated that it is geared to kill at great distances from its point of origin. Nuclear war, except for the terrible atom bombs dropped on Japan towards the end of World War II, has not been activated even though the threat is always with us. Terrorism, hi-jackings and other acts of violence seem to have become a way of life as the world nears the 21st century.

At the same time, there have been many advances in the care of the sick, in knowledge and treatment of diseases, and the development in many parts of the world of a social conscience, which has led to the enlightened care of human beings by other human beings. This historical overview has only been intended as a backdrop for what follows, and is of necessity merely a framework into which to fit the development of medicine, and especially nursing.

Alongside the events already mentioned have been the continuous occurrence of natural disasters, earthquakes, volcanic eruptions, floods, droughts with the attending famine, shipwrecks, tidal waves, hurricanes, typhoons and torna-does, and as man has developed his technology, massive train, mine and aircraft disasters are common phenomena. Due to the much larger population of the world, the numbers affected by these disasters continue to rise. Man has not yet been able to control natural disasters, but only to predict some of them to a limited degree. Despite all the technological advances he has not been able to harness the weather either.

5.2 Social changes

Ever since neolithic times, when man first learned how to cultivate the soil, the overwhelming majority of the population of the world has been occupied with agriculture. The development of mechanised farming has, however, resulted in this rural mode of existence coming to an end, bringing about significant changes in the way of life of the people of the world (5:164). In addition the effect of a gross population explosion must be considered, and it becomes clear that man is caught up in social change to which he will have to adapt. Social and economic change is occurring at breakneck speed and the future of mankind appears to be in the balance.

The knowledge explosion and the continual development of computer science also pose questions. As machines become more sophisticated, fewer men are needed to do more work. The result has been gross unemployment, shorter working hours, and a great deal of leisure time, which man does not put to constructive use. All these aspects hold potential health problems, mental as well as physical.

The period from 1800 onwards was characterised by the arousal of social conscience among people as a whole. It has already been pointed out that John Howard started a campaign designed to reform prisons. He did the same for hospitals.

Elizabeth Fry (1780-1845), a devout Quaker, was appalled by the squalor and depravity in prisons and did much to bring this to the notice of the public, whereby she aroused the conscience of the population as a whole. Her contribution to nursing reform will be discussed in section 5.4.7.

At the beginning of this period there was a very high mortality rate, one child in every three dying before the age of six. The evils of the industrial revolution, slums, overcrowding, poor sanitation, unhygienic conditions, ill-ventilated and badly lit overcrowded factories, long hours of work (14-18 hours a day) and the exploitation of women and child labour continued.

In 1802 an Act for the preservation of the health and morals of apprentices and others employed in cotton and other factories was passed in the English Parliament. Gradually the sense of social responsibility of mill-owners and the population generally began to be stirred. Pioneers in the work of reform were Thomas Cranfield (1766-1838) who began to work among slum children in Southwark, London in 1798 (5:28).

Authors of this period who did much to point out the current appalling social conditions included the poets Thomas Hood (*Song of the shirt*, 1834) and Elizabeth Barrett Browning (*The cry of the children*, 1844), and writers such as Mrs Frances Trollope (*Michael Armstrong, the factory boy*, 1840), Disraeli (*Sybil*, 1845), Mrs Elizabeth Gaskell (*Mary Barton*, 1848; *North and South*, 1889), Charles Kingsley (*Yeast*, 1848; *Alton Locke*, 1850), Charlotte Brontë (*Shirley*, 1849) and Charles Dickens (*Hard times*, 1854). These writers all contributed to bringing the appalling conditions to the notice of the public at large.

Cholera was the most devastating disease of the 19th century, with severe outbreaks occurring in 1832, 1849 and 1866 (8:183). Special places for the care of cholera-sufferers were set up in Exeter (England) and New York, among other places. The general unhygienic living standards must have contributed to these bad epidemics.

At the beginning of this period women were ascribed low social status. Their opportunities for education were extremely limited, but the mid 19th century saw the emergence of a movement for the recognition of the rights of women as human beings and the need for opportunities beyond basic education and entry into professions such as medicine and law.

Being a woman was a distinct disadvantage to those wishing to fulfil any but the traditional role of wife and mother. The educational backwater in which women found themselves also made it extremely difficult for nursing, which was and still is a predominantly female profession, to emerge and take its rightful place among its related professions. In spite of all this, many famous women fulfilled their aspirations. Elizabeth Blackwell, the first female medical doctor, graduated from the Geneva Medical College, New York, in 1849, after overcoming many difficulties to be accepted for study.

When one realises that secondary school education for girls in Britain only became established in the 1850s, girls were allowed to sit for the Cambridge local examinations in 1864 and London University admitted women to degree study only in 1874, then the difficulty of finding 'educated' women to train as nurses becomes clear.

As from 1861 women's colleges were established in America. In many countries women's education only developed after World War I and is still poorly developed in some of the Third World countries.

The social change that brought about general education for most girls and women was momentous. In countries where this has not yet been achieved, the nursing profession lags behind other professions and has not yet reached its full potential.

Throughout all this time, health care has lengthened man's lifespan, or at least the length of life reached by many people, and the worst infections which had been such prolific killers, were conquered. This has led to an ageing population, in the Western world at least, which has in turn resulted in more old people in the community and more social change. For example, it has become necessary to provide accommodation and a special form of health and social care for this increasingly growing group of people. Many of them are also caught up in economic problems as the value of their pensions and savings diminish due to economic factors such as inflation.

From this it should be clear that any form of social change has health implications which must always be borne in mind when taking the broad context of nursing history into consideration.

5.3 Scientific and medical changes

Nursing has been tremendously affected by the enormous developments that have taken place in science, medicine and surgery since 1800. As surgery became more generally available and its scope increased as a result of increased knowledge of human anatomy and physiology, the need for more better prepared, intelligent nurses increased. The introduction of antiseptic and aseptic practices, anaesthesia which has evolved very sophisticated techniques, and advances in medication and the medical management of disease also required better trained nurses. A willing worker, ignorant of 'what was going on' and only able to do what she was told to do, no longer met the changing health care needs. 'Soothing the fevered brow' was no longer enough. The emergence of modern nursing had its origins in the need to meet new demands.

A few of the scientific and medical advances which changed the face of health care and of the people who brought about such changes will be highlighted in the following sections.

5.3.1 The development of the stethoscope

In 1819, the French physician René Theophile Hyacinthe Laënnec (1781-

1826) invented the instrument which could be used to listen to the sounds of the respiratory, cardio-vascular and gastro-intestinal systems, as well as the heartbeat of the foetus in the uterus. Before this first stethoscope was devised (Greek *stethos* – breast; *skopos* – watcher), which was little more than a simple tube, the only way of hearing such sounds was by putting the listener's ear over the chest. This practice was not always approved by sufferers and their families, apart from considerations such as hygiene.

Laënnec was particularly interested in the 'white plague', tuberculosis, and in 1819 published his work *De l'auscultation mediaté*, which revolutionised the study of diseases of the chest (8:185,186; 32:3159,5109). Ironically, Laënnec himself died of tuberculosis. The stethoscope, which had such simple beginnings, has today become a very sophisticated instrument indeed.

5.3.2 Theory of heredity

Gregor Johan Mendel (1822-1884) was an Austrian Augustinian monk, whose study of plants and in particular edible sweet peas, led him to the conclusion that there was some natural law of inheritance. He formulated laws of heredity, bringing into use the terms *dominant* and *recessive* characteristics (32:3617,3618). His work formed the basis for the science of genetics, which has grown rapidly in the past two or three decades. Selective breeding of animals and of plants resistant to certain diseases and those producing better food yields, all emanated from his work.

5.3.3 The development of anaesthesia

The existence of certain substances such as opium and mandragora and large quantities of wine that could procure some insensitivity to pain has been known for centuries.

In 1800 Humphry Davy (1778-1829) suggested the use of nitrous oxide, or 'laughing gas', which had already been isolated in 1766 by Joseph Priestly as an anaesthetic. At the beginning of the 19th century the use of *ether* was introduced for this purpose. By 1847 ether was used in England and America generally (32:207,208).

In November 1847 Sir James Simpson introduced *chloroform* as an anaesthetic. Queen Victoria gave respectability to the use of anaesthesia in obstetrics by consenting to be anaesthetised for the birth of her seventh child, Princess Louise, later Duchess of Argyll. An interesting health fact that might be mentioned here is that Prince Albert, the husband of Queen Victoria, died in 1861 of typhoid fever, something extremely rare 100 years later.

Anaesthetics have come a long way since those early days, and can be administered in so many ways and in such different circumstances that it is now possible for the most complicated surgery to be carried out with comparative safety, even on 'bad risk' patients. Consequently, surgery has benefited greatly, and as a result the functions of the nurse have become even more complicated. However, she has never lost her humane, caring, person-to-person role, which is the very essence of nursing.

5.3.4 Antisepsis and asepsis

With the development of anaesthesia came the ability to perform surgery on persons who could be rendered insensitive to pain for the duration of the operation.

In the first half of the 19th century, however, 'wound infection very frequently complicated operations, and led to disaster in cases which might otherwise have been successfully treated' (22:267). Innumerable women also died in childbirth of puerperal sepsis. The high death rate in surgical wards of hospitals was a distressing fact for which no cause was known.

Ignaz Semmelweiss, a Hungarian obstetrician, came to the conclusion that the infection was conveyed from the autopsy room to the patients by dirty hands and instruments, and gave orders that hands were to be thoroughly washed and that wards were to be cleaned with calcium chloride. Despite a dramatic drop in the death rate, Semmelweiss was ridiculed by his colleagues and lost his post. He expanded on his theories and work in Hungary. His published work *Die Aetiologie, der Begriff und die Prophylaxis des Kinderbettfiebers* (1861) was not well written, and despite the valuable facts it contained, was neglected (22:267,268).

Louis Pasteur (1822-1895) was a French chemist and bacteriologist who discovered the micro-organism causing fermentation while working on the 'diseases' of beer, wine and vinegar, and developed 'pasteurisation' for the killing thereof. He did a great deal of other work on diseases of silkworms and chickens, as well as on cholera, anthrax and rabies and discovered that it was possible to attenuate disease-producing organisms and to use the serum for immunisation (32:4202). His work on micro-organisms had important implications for antiseptic and aseptic techniques that were developed.

Joseph Lister (1827-1912), a Scottish surgeon, was deeply concerned with the large number of deaths due to wound infection. Pasteur's work was known to him and he believed that either the micro-organisms which Pasteur had described or other similar ones could enter wounds and cause 'infection'. He felt that it was necessary to kill the bacteria already in wounds, and to apply dressings which were impregnated with some substance which would kill micro-organisms. It had not yet been proved that micro-organisms caused disease, but he insisted on meticulous cleanliness in his wards and the instruments used, and started using phenol to kill organisms which he believed were the culprits. Lister also introduced carbolised catgut for suturing. He is regarded as the founder of antiseptic principles, and his work, because of its striking success in reducing wound infection, changed the whole nature of surgery (32:3342).

Antisepsis, the killing of micro-organisms, was followed by *asepsis*, which was not aimed at the killing of micro-organisms, but at excluding them entirely from the operating theatre, and from wound dressings.

Pasteur had introduced heat for preventing fermentation. This was carried a step further by the German Ernst von Bergmann (1837-1907) who introduced the sterilisation of dressings through the use of steam in 1866.

In 1890 the American WS Halstead (1852-1922) introduced the use of sterile rubber gloves into surgery (32:268,269).

Of particular relevance to the student of the history of nursing is that the Fliedners at Kaiserwerth (section 5.4.3) were active during the period when all these medical developments were occurring, and that Florence Nightingale went to the Crimea in 1854, where she established order in the barracks hospital at Scutari through the application of cleanliness and hygiene, and effective administration (section 5.4.4).

Johannes Müller (1801-1858) laid the foundations of scientific medicine in Germany, while Joka B Henle (1809-1885), the discoverer of the renal tubules which bear his name, was among the first to maintain that micro-organisms caused infectious disease.

5.3.5 Other important scientific and medical advances

Due to the continual improvement in microscopes, the study of pathology progressed rapidly and broadened to include pathophysiology. Great advances were contstantly being made in the field of microbiology, not only in relation to wound infection, but to disease causation generally. The existence of filterable viruses was demonstrated.

However, microscopes were for a long time not sophisticated enough to enable man to 'see' viruses. That had to wait till the 20th century, which saw the development of electronic microscopy.

The organism causing bubonic plague was isolated in 1894 by GAE Yersin and Kitasato, working independently.

Albert Calmette (1863-1933) discovered a protective serum against snakebite and the BCG vaccine against tuberculosis. Elia Metchikoff (1845-1916) was the first to shed light on the essential nature of the infective process and immunisation, and is famous for his work on phagocytosis.

Robert Koch (1843-1910) carried on Pasteur's work and laid down his 'postulates', a famous set of rules which must be obeyed if it is to be proved that a specific organism is responsible for a specific disease. These postulates (22:276) include the following

☐ the organism must always be found in a given disease

☐ the organism must not be found in other diseases or in health

☐ the organism must be cultivated artificially and reproduce the given disease after the inoculation of a pure culture into a susceptible animal

☐ the organism must be recoverable from the animal so inoculated.

Following these postulates, Koch isolated and cultured the *mycobacterium tuberculosis* in 1882.

Emil von Behring and Baron Shibasaburo Kitasato published papers in 1890 proclaiming the discovery of antitoxins and their use in passive immunisation against tetanus and diphtheria.

Paul Ehrlich (1854-1915) was the founder of modern chemotherapy and immunology. He formulated the hypothesis that certain dyes had an affinity for specific tissues and could thus select specific micro-organisms. He developed *salvarsan* for the treatment of syphilis. Fritz Schaudinn (1871-1906) discovered the causative organism of this disease, and August von Wassermann (1866-1925) devised a diagnostic test. Julius Morgenroth (1871-1924), Richard Pfeiffer (1858-1945) and others made important contributions to the field of immunology including immune bodies, complement athermo-labile substance and complement fixation tests, antigens, opsonins and auto-immune conditions.

Insect vectors as transmitters of disease, particularly tropical disease, received attention.

Patrick Manson (1844-1922) the 'father' of modern tropical medicine, showed that a minute parasitic worm found in the blood of humans suffering from elephantiasis was transmitted to man by the mosquito *culex fagitans*. It is interesting to note that Susruta's writings had suggested the possibility of insect transmission of disease more than one thousand years before. In Cuba Finlay (1832-1915) and later in 1900 Walter Reed (Panama Canal), showed the part played by the *aedes aegypti* mosquito in the spread of yellow fever.

Laveran of Algiers isolated the plasmodium of malaria in 1880 and Ronald Ross showed the part played by the *anopheles* mosquito in its transmission in 1898. *Rikettsiae* as a cause of various diseases, including Rocky Mountain spotted fever and typhus, were also identified in the early 20th century.

With the development of the electron microscope in the 1930s, it became possible to see and identify viruses. Jonas Salk introduced a vaccine against poliomyelitis in 1954, followed by the attenuated oral Sabin vaccine for the same disease.

To combat more general infections, chemical substances were developed. Prontosil was developed by Gerhard Domack in 1935, while the sulphonamides (M&B 693), sulphapyridine, and others were introduced from 1938 onwards. From this beginning sprung a vast armentarium of effective medications against a variety of infections. Alexander Fleming (1881-1955) discovered the effect of the fungus *penicillium notatum* on a culture of staphylococci, and *penicillin* was eventually isolated in 1940.

Strains of organisms resistant to drugs also developed, inspiring further work in the field, and other antibiotics as well as variants to penicillin continued to prove effective against disease (22:270-282).

At the same time as drugs were being developed, an occurrence of equal importance to the progress of medical knowledge and practice took place, namely the emergence of the science of radiology.

Wilhelm Konrad Roentgen (1845-1923) discovered the properties of rays which he named X-rays in 1895. This discovery revolutionised diagnostic practices and later also led to the therapeutic application of radiation to malignant tumours. Radio-opaque substances for outlining internal organs were also developed to aid diagnosis (22:284,286).

It was the French physicist Henri Bequerel who discovered natural radioactivity of uranium in 1903 (22:287), and the possibility of photographing what was shown by X-rays instead of simple direct viewing.

In 1898 Pierre Curie and his wife Marya Sklodovska (Marya was Polish; she was known as Marie in France) isolated polonium and discovered radium (22:287). An outcome of these beginnings was the discovery of artificial radioactivity by Irène Curie and her husband Frédéric Joliot in 1931 (22:287), and the development of radioactive isotopes for treatment and diagnosis.

The first corneal grafting was performed in 1883, while the first human kidney transplant was performed in 1950 by RH Lawler.

Between 1919 and 1923 insulin was prepared and injected into humans for the treatment of diabetes mellitus, America produced the first 'iron lung' respirator, electronic hearing aids were developed and an electroencephalograph became reality through work originally done in Germany.

Between 1929 and 1938 an artificial cardiac pacemaker was developed in the United States of America, blood grouping and blood transfusions became standard practice and the RH blood factor was discovered, also in the United States of America. In Italy electroconvulsive therapy was introduced for the first time.

Between 1939 and 1944 streptomycin, which made a great difference to the treatment of tuberculosis, was first produced in the United States of America, followed by the introduction of drugs such as isoniazid, rifampin, ethambutol and para-aminosalicylic acid. New drugs were constantly tested and used as their efficacy was proved. During this period the first kidney machine was developed in the Netherlands, while from 1945 to 1956 the operation for the treatment of babies with Fallot's tetralogy and later other heart ailments was developed. A clear plastic corneal lens was manufactured, and a commercial synthetic process for the production of cortisone in the USA, as well as the first 'heart-lung' machine, was evolved.

The first synthetic progestin was another addition to the medical armentarium. The first successful cardiopulmonary bypass operation was carried out in the USA and the first successful use of an artificial heart valve for humans was inserted during this time. In 1953 the discovery of the structure of DNA was made by two scientists at Cambridge University.

During the period from 1957 to 1982 so many advances, new discoveries and developments took place that it is difficult to even attempt to select the most important since importance is also a relative concept. A few will be mentioned, but it must be realised that these only give an indication of the fast rate of change on the medical scene.

Oral and intra-uterine contraception became a reality, which made it possible to control the population increase from 1960 onwards. However, its universal application and acceptance has, despite the tremendous overpopulation of the world, still not become a reality. The first successful cardiac pacemaker was implanted in the USA and open-heart surgery has become commonplace. So too has renal dialysis, with the result that patients often have home dialysis units.

The first human heart transplant was performed by Dr Christiaan Barnard at Groote Schuur Hospital in Cape Town in 1967. Although the recipient of the first human heart, Louis Washkansky, did not survive very long, many more have since been performed successfully. The first artificial human heart, used on a Dr B Clark in the USA in 1982, was not very successful, and experiments are still being carried out.

Genetic engineering has become a possibility following the successful synthesising of a gene, the fundamental unit of heredity. Human ova have been fertilised outside the body and then implanted into the uterus of the mother who then gives birth to a baby in the normal way (in vitro fertilisation).

Ultrasonic scanning has replaced the use of X-rays in many instances, so that monitoring of the development of a foetus can be carried out without the danger of radiation to mother and baby. It has also many other medical uses.

One of the most dramatic changes that has occurred is in the field of nervous and mental diseases, which seem to become more prevalent in modern society.

The first attempts to classify psychiatric diseases were made in the 18th century, and at the same time restraint, starvation, close confinement and other violent methods of 'treatment' began to be supplanted by more humane treatment.

Philippe Pinel (1758-1828), a French physician, was appointed to the asylum at Bicêtre in 1793, and was the first to release patients who had been chained. He continued his work at the Saltpêtrière in Paris. Jean Martin Charcot (1825-1893) was a great French neurologist under whom the Saltpêtrière became the centre of neurology.

Sigmund Freud (1856-1939) studied neuroanatomy and neuropathology in Vienna and at the Saltpêtrière. On return to Vienna in 1886, he initiated modern psychoanalytic methods. Carl Gustav Jung (1875-1961), Alfred Adler (1870-1937) and Otto Rank (1884-1939) continued his work although they modified his basic theories (22:294-297).

Neurosurgery also made great strides but the great breakthrough in the treatment of mental illness came with the development of medications such as the psychotropic drugs which have powerful effects on mental disturbances, while leaving intelligence and awareness unimpaired. This has enabled the early discharge of acutely disturbed patients and their successful re-integration into the community.

The pace at which new developments take place, has continued to increase. The consequent increase in the skills needed by the nurse to monitor patients on various machines, to deal with life-threatening emergencies, to defibrillate when necessary, to give cardiopulmonary resuscitation where applicable, to recognise the iatrogenic effects of drug therapy and take appropriate action, to stitch wounds and administer intravenous therapy, all need a level of knowledge and skill not dreamed of at the beginning of the period under discussion, a mere 190 years since 1880. At the same time emphasis should still be placed on the *human* contact role of the nurse as a human being, treating other human beings with humanity and compassion.

Great advances were also made in the field of community health with the development of waterborne sewerage, safe water and food supplies, and the disposal of refuse. This has taken time, but at last areas which were grossly polluted, such as the River Thames in London, are once more stocked with fish. Smokefree zones in some cities have also ensured that some air is relatively unpolluted. The preservation of wild life and natural flora and fauna and the achievement of an ecological balance is constantly striven for.

Unfortunately there are still too many areas in our world where the hygienic standards and services to the population leave much to be desired. Man has the necessary knowhow, but does not always apply this knowledge. This is due to the great number of different factors that are involved, economics playing a large part.

5.4 The development of nursing

This was one of the most momentous periods in the history of the development of nursing. In the beginning nursing had not attained recognition and had not been 'rediscovered' as a profession. It had not yet obtained general respectability or acceptance as a suitable occupation for well-bred or 'respectable' women, beyond the religious sisters.

The duties of those who were supposedly devoted to the care of the sick were not undertaken by women of much standing or even decent behaviour, with the exception of care given in the home by the women of the household. The pattern, especially in many English hospitals, was not very edifying. In contrast, those hospitals run by the religious sisterhoods who nursed because it was their calling or 'vocation' to care for the sick, may not have been remarkable for their standard of nursing knowledge, but their conduct was unquestionable.

In civilian life the quality of many women used for this work must have been appalling, as were the conditions under which they were expected to work. In the London Hospital, for instance, day staff had to be on duty at 6 am in summer and at 7 am in winter, and had to be in bed by 11 pm every night. They had no days off and no holidays, and their tasks included cleaning the wards, the pewter and utensils, keeping the patients neat and clean and giving out medicines.

Records show that drunkenness, thieving, selling of food to patients, and trying in other ways to make money out of patients were commonplace. The pay was a princely sum of £14 (R28) per annum and they had to sleep in ward units. Many women were elderly, with doubtful 'pasts', and could not earn their living any other way.

There were however exceptions and devoted care was indeed being given by certain women, even in the degenerate state to which much nursing had been reduced (36: article 10).

As has already been stated, knowledgeable, intelligent persons were required to meet the ever-increasing needs of patients and the medical team. As

knowledge about disease and treatment increased, more and more sophisticated diagnostic methods developed and surgery became possible in cases
where it had previously been unthinkable, the demand, indeed the absolute
necessity for a body of skilled, knowledgeable, intelligent nurses became an
urgent necessity.

It must not be forgotten that medical education also underwent dramatic
changes to meet changing times. The preceptor-apprentice system of medical
education, with lack of uniform laws regarding medical qualifications, practice
and licensure was in force. The change in the nature of medicine, with the
physician needing more information about signs and symptoms in order to
treat the patient effectively has brought a need for continuous, detailed
observation by persons knowledgeable about sick people, besides their need for
purely physical care. This need is met by nurses.

As medicine evolved into a scientific profession, so did nursing. This was a
lengthy process, hampered by the social position of women and the overall lack
of general education. These limitations were overcome due to a few far-sighted
people and institutions who recognised the needs for better nursing care.

It is a generally held belief that nursing began with Florence Nightingale,
which the reader of this history will by now have realised, simply is not true.
However, that she had a tremendous influence on modern nursing, is an
indisputable fact. Her contributions as well as those of a few others will now
be discussed in more detail.

5.4.1 Franz May

In 1781 Franz May of Mannheim in Germany persuaded some of the
authorities who were responsible for the running of hospitals to provide a series
of lectures to successive groups of 'nursing attendants'. This effectively
constituted the beginning of the training of secular nurses in hospitals and took
place some 50 years before the establishment of the Nightingale School. It was
in Germany that the first integrated course of theory and practice was
organised, leading to certification. This was a major step in the development
of nursing, from care given by people with no real knowledge of what they were
doing to that given by people who had formal instruction in the skills they were
practising.

Several other schools, which all added to the emergence of nursing as a highly
regarded profession, were established in Germany between 1782 and 1815.
This was a result of a general upsurge of interest in the health of the people as
a whole, and the enlightened attitude of doctors in the Reformation period
towards their patients. Dr Valentine Seaman also gave a series of lectures to
nurses in a New York hospital in 1798.

5.4.2 Bishop Grégoire

In 1819 Bishop Grégoire appealed for a system of teaching nurses in France.
The medical profession also pressed for nursing nuns to be taught medical
subjects in addition to their purely religious instruction. This led to nursing

nuns of the religious orders receiving at least some form of instruction in nursing and related subjects.

5.4.3 The Fliedners of Kaiserwerth

A Lutheran minister, Pastor Theodor Fliedner (1800-1864), and his wife Frederika Münster founded the *Kaiserwerth Institute for the Training of Deaconesses* in 1836, thus contributing to the restoration of the ancient religious order of deaconesses. This institute had training centres for teachers in nursery, elementary, and vocational and high schools. They also ran a kindergarten and a hospital which served as a training school for nurses. Although the deaconesses took no vows except a promise to 'work for Christ', high standards of behaviour were expected from them. The deaconesses were provided with a permanent home from which they worked, not only in the hospital, but in private homes and almshouses. Frederika Fliedner died in 1842, and when Pastor Fliedner remarried, Caroline Fliedner carried on with the work of nursing instruction. Florence Nightingale visited Kaiserwerth, and its influence spread to America with the founding of the first Protestant Church hospital in America at Pittsburgh in 1849 (8:203,204).

5.4.4 Florence Nightingale (1820-1910)

This young lady was the daughter of wealthy parents, born in Florence, from which she received her name.

In her early teens Florence Nightingale visited the sick poor in her neighbourhood, as was the custom among the women of well-to-do families in the Victorian era. She also cared for a sick grandmother, and visited the sick of the village of Wellow for many years. On reaching the age of 20 she expressed the desire to train as a nurse, but her parents, well aware of the poor conditions existing in hospitals at the time, refused to allow this. During the course of her travels she visited hospitals in Germany, France, Belgium and Italy, in 1850 spending two weeks at Kaiserwerth. She returned for a further three months in 1851.

Florence Nightingale herself always denied that she had been 'trained' at Kaiserwerth, writing in 1897 that 'the nursing was nil, and the hygiene horrible' (31:70). She also spent some time with the Sisters of Charity in their hospital in the Maison de la Providence in Paris in 1853.

Her father eventually gave her an allowance of £500 (±R2000) a year which made Florence financially independent. She was appointed superintendent of the *Institution for the Care of Sick Gentlewomen in Distressed Circumstances*, and there showed her genius for organisation and administration. Reform was difficult for although the need for a better type of nurse was obvious, none existed. This convinced her that before any form of nursing reform could be embarked on, the following prerequisites should be met.

> [A] training school capable of producing a supply of respectable, reliable, qualified nurses must be brought into existence. Her first task must be to produce a new type of nurse (31:91).

A cholera epidemic in 1854 in London gave her further experience of prevailing conditions in health and nursing care.

When the Crimean War broke out, her career reached its turning point. She visited the region and was appalled by hospital conditions there: hospitals were filled to overflowing, and had insufficient drugs, sanitary conveniences, bedding and feeding arrangements. Cholera broke out, and added to the already high battle casualties. There were no 'Sisters of Charity' as the French had – in fact, there were no nurses to look after the British troops who were ill or wounded at all.

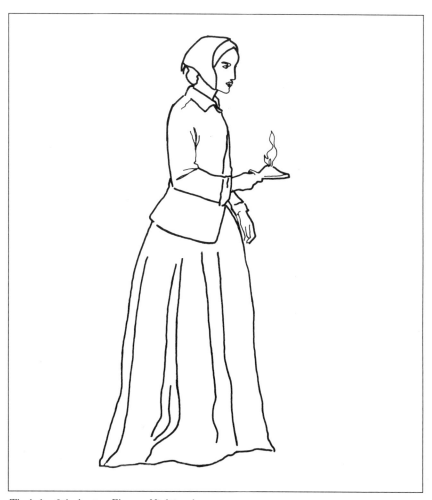

The lady of the lamp – Florence Nightingale

Sidney Herbert, the Secretary of War, arranged for Florence Nightingale to go out to Scutari, which was across the strait from Constantinople (now Istanbul), with a party of 30 nurses, as superintendent of the female nursing establishment of the English general military hospitals in Turkey. Her party consisted of 14 experienced lay nurses and 24 members of religious institutions.

The conditions of their engagement were extremely strict and Florence Nightingale was in sole charge.

She encountered many difficulties and much opposition at first. There were between 3 000 and 4 000 sick and wounded, the conditions were indescribable, there was no equipment, and not surprisingly the mortality rate was 42 per cent. Florence Nightingale's organising ability, her genius with statistics and her capacity for analysing a situation and instituting reform were given an opportunity to be put to good use. She was an intellectual who had influential connections at home and was capable of putting facts on paper in a clear, logical way. She gathered and analysed data in a scientific manner.

Within six months she transformed the hospital at Scutari, reducing the death rate from 42 per cent to 2 per cent.

Although her name is remembered in nursing, her influence was much wider, for she was a hygienist, a statistician, a writer and an efficient administrator who was responsible for many reforms besides those in nursing.

As a result of her work in the Crimea and the fund that was collected to honour her (the Nightingale Fund of £45 000 – a great deal of money in those days), the Nightingale School for Nurses was established at St Thomas' Hospital in London in 1860. Mrs Wardroper was chosen to take charge.

This was the beginning of modern nursing education in England, and its influence spread throughout the world. Florence Nightingale's writings are most illuminating and can be read with profit today. One of the passages from her work which could well bear quoting is 'Nursing is helping people to live and training is to teach the nurse how to help the patient to live' (8:219).

The aim of the Nightingale School was threefold: to train 'matrons' who could organise hospitals and train others, to train hospital nurses who could supervise the untrained and to train district nurses for the sick poor (8:218).

The selection of applicants was very strict, as was the code of behaviour. Due to this, nursing attained respectability and subsequently educated women from the upper and middle strata of society were attracted to nursing. A nurses' home provided a 'safe' haven for probationers, so that no breath of scandal could touch the young ladies in training.

Florence Nightingale envisaged the training as being suitable for any intelligent girl with the right attitude, but the scheme tended to attract those from the upper classes (1:73). At first ordinary probationers, who paid no fee and received free maintenance, did a two-year training course while 'lady' probationers, who paid for their training, did a one-year training. Eventually a two-year period became standard. As early as 1867 a ward sister received money from the Nightingale Fund for her part in assisting in the training of students, in addition to what she was paid by the hospital. Thus the teaching role of the 'ward sister' was established early on in modern training patterns, something that many registered nurses of today tend to forget.

5.4.5 The training school at Lausanne

Florence Nightingale's training school at St Thomas' Hospital was preceded by a school for training of 'lay nurses' at Lausanne in Switzerland in 1859. These nurses were not attached in any way to religious congregations where nursing care was undertaken by nuns, oblates, deaconesses and the like.

5.4.6 Training in other countries

The first organised training of nurses in America occurred when schools of nursing were established in New York, New Haven and Boston in 1873. At first the training was based on the Nightingale pattern, but later developed its own style.

5.4.6.1 The religious nursing orders

The early part of the 19th century saw the religious nursing orders taking a form of organised nursing to the New World. Elizabeth Bayley Seton (1774-1821), a widow, began the Sisters of Charity at Emmitsburg in 1809, eventually uniting with the Sisters of Charity of St Vincent de Paul. Other Roman Catholic nursing orders which were established in America included the Irish Sisters of Charity, the Sisters of Mercy and the Sisters of the Holy Cross. Religious sisters staffed the larger, better run hospitals during the American Civil War (8:199-201).

The Anglican sisterhoods became established in England in about 1848, using religious sisters as well as deaconesses for hospital and community work. Their work was extended to the United States and also to Africa.

The community of St Michael and All Angels, established in Bloemfontein, to which Sister Henrietta belonged was one of these Anglican orders.

Deaconesses from Protestant churches, such as the Methodist Church and others, also played a part in the development of nursing and its spread from Europe to other parts of the world.

5.4.7 Elizabeth Fry (1780-1845)

She was a staunch Quaker and most noted as a prison reformer. However, she was interested in all social problems. As a young woman she visited the sick in their homes, as was the custom of the time for the young women of better-class families (her father was a banker). She also visited Kaiserwerth and, much impressed by the work of the deaconesses, intended to form a similar nursing system when she returned to England. However, her prison reform activities prevented her from giving this much attention, although she did found a Society of Protestant Sisters of Charity at Bishopsgate, with the help of a sister and daughter, which later became the Institution of Nursing Sisters. These selected, supervised women received some hospital training at Guy's Hospital, but they were mainly prepared for the private nursing of the sick of all classes and to do welfare work. It was not an entirely successful venture (32:2281; 1:23,24; 8:202).

5.4.8 Agnes Jones

Together with 12 nurses, Agnes Jones, a pupil of Florence Nightingale, organised the nursing of male inmates of the Brownlow Hill Institution, a workhouse in Liverpool in 1865.

Although successful at first, this venture suffered a tremendous setback by the death of Miss Jones from typhus, which she caught in the course of her work. Nevertheless much needed workhouse reform had been started.

5.4.9 Dorothea Lynde Dix (1802-1887)

She is famous for her pioneer work in the reform of the care of the mentally ill in America.

5.4.10 Mrs Bedford Fenwick

Mrs Bedford Fenwick is remembered as having founded the Royal British Nurses' Association in 1887 and for her fight for state registration. She was a friend of Sister Henrietta Stockdale, but was bitterly opposed by Florence Nightingale in her attempt to get state registration for nurses in England, which was only achieved in 1902 for midwives and in 1919 for nurses. The Cape Colony obtained state registration in 1891 through the efforts of Sister Henrietta Stockdale.

Mrs Bedford Fenwick was also the founder of the *International Council of Nurses* in 1899. The first meeting of the Council, duly constituted, took place in 1901. This was the first professional women's organisation on an international level and Sister Henrietta was a member of the founding committee.

5.4.11 Nursing associations in other countries

The formation of the International Council of Nurses (ICN), which only granted membership to national associations, led to the formation of such associations in other parts of the world. Examples of these are the Canadian Association in 1908, the American Nursing Association in 1911, and the South African Trained Nurses' Association, later the South African Nursing Association, in 1914. The movement spread to other British colonies and later independent African states, to Germany, Denmark, Sweden, France, Belgium and many others.

5.4.12 Nursing education

The form that this has taken has varied from the early patterns and includes the Nightingale system (with many modifications), some from the American system, some from the Motherhouse system and some from the Continental system. Many of them have been adapted to meet the needs of the different countries and have automatically been modified by the level of education of the potential students. Some form of registration of basic qualifications, and in many cases of peer group control of the profession, is widespread.

Because nursing is a dynamic profession, nursing education is always undergoing change and modification.

Nursing education has also reached university level and many countries now have a corps of graduate nurses who make a valuable contribution to nursing care in their communities.

The increasing specialisation in medicine has led to specialisation in nursing, with post-registration specialist nursing courses being provided further to educate registered nurses to meet the needs of the community for specialised care.

The field of nursing education has also led to the need for trained nurse educators to teach and guide the neophytes in the profession, and the extension of nurses into nursing administration posts has required trained nurse administrators.

Midwifery has become more and more complex and specialised, and often requires education beyond that obtained at basic level. The needs of the community for 'specialist' nurses must also be met in many other fields, such as occupational health nursing. Psychiatric nursing is also demanding in-creased skills and oncology nursing, geriatric nursing, and genetic counselling all make their demands on nursing education. Space-age medicine has already made an impact and will continue to do so. Sport medicine is another growing field.

5.4.13 Research in nursing

As modern nursing has emerged from the Dark Ages and become an organised profession, it has become necessary to take a look at the profession, to research the needs of the consumers of nursing care, and of its practitioners, and then to make the necessary adjustments to eliminate problem areas and to meet the needs that have been identified. This area of nursing has a tremendous scope for expansion.

Nursing remains rooted in *service* and the search for new knowledge and skills must always take into account the purpose for which it exists, namely, the *care* of people in need, which makes nursing unique.

5.5 Factors in history which have influenced the development of nursing

At this stage it is appropriate to look at various factors in history which have affected the development of nursing and nursing history through the ages. The history of nursing would be incomplete without the examination of the effects of certain social institutions and trends which have affected health care and the need for specific health care throughout the ages.

5.5.1 Religion

It must have become clear to those reading this text that religious beliefs and practices have been linked with health care from time immemorial.

Men have always held some belief in a force outside themselves which was considered to rule their destinies.

Belief in the powers of a supreme being or beings has been widespread throughout history. This was a form of religion. Religion has been defined as a human recognition of a superhuman controlling power (41:1027). 'Religion' encompasses a wide range of beliefs from the 'magical powers' of inanimate objects such as charms, amulets and totem poles, to the worship of ancestors and a belief in the existence of spirits and gods who held the fate of human beings in their hands. These religious beliefs developed into a system of faith or a specific religion.

Because ill people needed help from 'outside', many magical practices developed to which sufferers were subjected. Sometimes empirical use of herbs and other medications developed which were beneficial to those seeking relief. Whatever the case, religions have throughout the ages influenced the way man lived his life, his work ethic and his attitudes and relationships.

Primitive cultures found the causes of disease difficult to understand. It was simple to see the effect of a sharp stone cutting the skin. External injuries were visible, therefore clear and understandable, but there was no logical obvious explanation for internal pain, coughing, fever or paralysis. But these things occurred and the 20th century nurse might have difficulty relating to health care without the benefit of modern scientific medicine and the uncertainty, fear and distress in the minds of primitive people. Yet we all know the effect of mind over the body, are acquainted with the occurrence of psycho-somatic diseases and know the comfort which patients receive from those who minister to their religious needs.

Medical practice had its origins in the belief that magic could prevent ill-health; magical powers were seen to be possessed by the shamans or witchdoctors of the time. Evil spirits were often believed to be attacking people and causing the symptoms of the evident disease. These evil spirits had to be appeased, encouraged to leave the bodies of those afflicted, or precautions had to be taken against people being attacked. The shamans developed all sorts of ritualistic procedures to ward off disease or to treat it when it occurred. This 'treatment' was based on the religious concepts of the times.

Ancestor worship was also practised and ill-health might be ascribed to failure to carry out required practices of worship. Since the ancestors were sacred, the human body, which had housed the spirit of the dead person who had now become an 'ancestor' was also sacred and could not be studied. This meant that medical knowledge did not develop. Herbal remedies which had proved effective by trial and error were used and the use of massage became general, perhaps developing from the belief that 'punishing' the body (by pummelling) also got rid of evil spirits which were tormenting it.

5.5.1.1 Temples and priest physicians

As societies became more sophisticated, the worship of the gods which were accepted in an area became concentrated in one specific place. This aspect has already been discussed when we were dealing with Greek culture. Those who were ill came or were brought to the place of worship of their God so that the priests could pray for a cure or help them to pacify gods who they believed were angry and had caused their disease.

Temples developed around the places of worship and resulted in a fixed community with their own priests and attendants. Because these priests also helped to treat the sick, they became known as priest physicians.

Many sick people stayed at the temples to receive treatment from the priest-physicians, and temple attendants had to assist in their care. These attendants were perhaps the first 'nurses' outside the nursing care given in the home by mothers and other members of the family and slaves who until then had cared for the sick, injured and helpless.

The effects of some widespread religions are discussed briefly.

5.5.1.2 Buddhism

This religion had its origins in the sixth century BCE with an Indian prince, *Siddhartha Guatama*, who became known as the 'Enlightened One'. Buddhism spread rapidly throughout India and to Burma, Ceylon, Thailand, China, Mongolia, Korea and Japan. It even reached the Tatars of South Eastern Russia (32). Buddhism states that pain and suffering exist and that man is doomed to suffer. As long as man strives for himself and for the pleasures of his life, he will suffer. This interest in his own good and striving for the good things in life must be overcome before pain and suffering can be conquered.

This teaching saw disease to be caused by straying from the correct course set for man to gain enlightenment, and was therefore a just punishment which had to be endured. This belief was not conducive to the development of medical knowledge or of nursing.

In later times Buddhism largely disappeared from India, to be replaced by Hinduism, even though it still flourishes in other parts of the world.

5.5.1.3 Hinduism

This is a comprehensive term used to designate the social customs and religious beliefs of the majority of people in present-day India.

Hinduism developed in India between the fourth and fifth centuries BCE. It has many different important gods, including Brahma, Shiva, Vishnu and Krishna. Brahma is the supreme being in the Hindu pantheon, many other gods being seen as manifestations of him. Brahma cannot be clearly delineated.

The Brahman 'scriptures or writings', the *Vedas*, were believed to be a divine gift from Brahma. These books were the historical documents of India and their doctrines were presented in the form of hymns, prayers and teachings (9:59). The *Vedas* and commentaries on them discussed, *inter alia*, the medicinal use of herbs and the use of incantations to treat physical ills. Due to these being 'sacred' books, the religious aspects of Hindu 'medical' practice became obvious.

5.5.1.4 The Hebrew religion

The Hebrews were monotheistic, worshipping only one god. The high priests of this religion practised as priest-physicians and health inspectors, basing their practices on the Mosaic Code, the law given to Moses by God.

This 'law' was an organised set of rules for the prevention of disease and the promotion of health. It included aspects of personal hygiene, female hygiene in relation to menstruation and childbirth, the slaughtering of animals for food, the disposal of refuse and human excreta and control of communicable diseases, including recognition, isolation, quarantine and disinfection. Again this was a 'divine order' and the religious rules affected health care in a broad sense.

5.5.1.5 The religion of the ancient Greeks

The ancient Greeks developed a special god of healing, Apollo, whose son Asklepios was the God of Medicine. Hygeia, the goddess of health, and Panacea, the goddess of medication, were daughters of Asklepios. A large temple dedicated to Asklepios was built at Epidauros and a medical centre grew up around the temple.

Hippocrates, generally known as the 'father of medicine', belonged to an Asklepiad family. The Asklepiades were an order of priests who were supposed to be descended from Asklepios and claimed a knowledge of medicine.

The *Hippocratic Oath*, which set a standard for medical ethics, commenced with the following words:

> I swear by Apollo, the healer, by Asklepios, by health and all the powers of healing, and call to witness all the gods and goddesses that I may keep this oath . . .

It was used to initiate men into the art and practice of medicine. Again the practice of medicine was clearly linked with religion.

5.5.1.6 Christianity

This religion exerted a great influence on health care since Christianity was largely concerned with the recognition of every man's human worth as an individual. Service to man was service to God.

Nursing as a separate entity began in the early Christian period. Before this time the care of the sick, except by those nearest and dearest to them, was entrusted to slaves. Christian service to the sick spread into the community; orders of deaconesses and monastic orders were established, and the nuns 'who took the veil' started an influence on nursing and nursing history that has endured to this day.

The Emperor Julian (c 331-363 CE) stated that the care given by Christians to the sick was one of the factors that made them enemies of the then powerful Roman gods.

The Protestant Reformation, a religious movement in Christianity, initially did a great deal of harm to medicine and nursing because of the destruction of monasteries and convents and their attached hospitals. The revival of the deaconess orders by the Protestant churches led to a renewed awareness of the care of the sick as a religious duty, and missions to all parts of the world opened up health care to many people as hospitals developed alongside evangelism. In Southern Africa it was the Christian missions that paved the way for the training of Black women as nurses.

5.5.2 Wars

It is a sad reflection on humanity that from the earliest times men have waged war with one another and still continue to do so.

The weapons of war, from the most primitive to the sophisticated modern weapons capable of destroying large numbers of non-combatants as well as soldiers, have inflicted wounds on casualties who have needed medical and nursing care.

In early times a wound that became infected was usually fatal. Today antibiotics help combat infection and modern surgical treatment can repair much of the damage inflicted on the human body or other techniques can supply functional prostheses.

Besides the deaths and destruction caused by enemy action, many armies have been defeated by epidemics which followed the breakdown of hygiene and sanitary practices. Often many more soldiers were killed by disease than by enemy action. The total war of modern times, where the destructive force is not only directed at the opposing soldiers, but also at the civilian population makes the spread of disease to bombed populations part of the reality of modern warfare.

In early times slaves looked after the sick and wounded soldiers during wartime, wars which were often fought far from the homes of the combatants. In their imperial conquests which spread over large parts of Europe, the Romans actually erected large, well-planned hospitals designed to care for the soldiers, sick and wounded during their campaigns abroad. Remember that it did not take only a few hours to travel from Britain to Rome, as is the case today, but many weeks of slow travel. Casualties could not be evacuated, they had to be cared for on the spot. The sick and wounded in these Roman army hospitals were tended by military personnel as well as slaves.

The *Crusades*, which were religious wars waged between 1095 and 1291 by Western Europeans in an attempt to regain the Holy Land from the Muslims, were on the whole unsuccessful. From a nursing point of view they led to the formation of well-organised military nursing orders to look after the Crusaders. The objectives of these orders were religious as well as military and their influence is seen in the combination of the religious component (nursing as a vocation) and military practices (the strict rules and military hierarchical structure in nursing) which came about in the nursing services which developed later. These military nursing orders included the Knights Hospitallers of St John of Jerusalem, the Knights of St Lazarus, and the Teutonic Knights. These orders built many fine hospitals and developed a good system of hospital administration. Although these hospitals were mainly constructed to care for the soldiers of the Crusades, they also cared for those who fell ill on their pilgrimages to the Holy Land.

Many nursing traditions which are still honoured today have their origins in military nursing, which dates back to the Crusades. These include the rigid etiquette that was followed by military orders, the rounds with the physicians and the physical pattern of nursing units, with a large ward for the less ill patients, side wards for the more seriously ill and cubicles for those in a critical state.

Despite these early developments resulting in the establishment of military nursing orders, military medicine, which aimed at treating sick as well as wounded soldiers, was slow to develop. It was only at the end of the eighteenth century that military medicine became part of the organisation of the army and a permanent medical corps, army hospitals and field medical casualty stations became a reality.

The Napoleonic wars finally brought disaster to the French nation, which lost large numbers of its force through disease. This event brought France to the realisation that there was a great need for really efficient medical care for soldiers during war time. The Crimean War did the same for the British when Florence Nightingale, working with a heterogeneous group of Catholic nuns, Anglican sisters and lay nurses, brought the death rate of those treated in Scutari down from 427 to 22 per thousand. This she achieved by sanitary reforms, serving proper diets, training orderlies and proper individual care. She fought a bitter battle to achieve these reforms and eventually established nursing as a respectable profession for which training was necessary.

The Crimean War and the experience Florence Nightingale gained because of it has moulded the pattern of modern nursing in no uncertain way. The American Civil War was another national disaster in which twice as many soldiers succumbed to disease as to battle wounds.

Disease has played a large part in military campaigns, malaria being one of the most serious of such diseases (39:24). For example in the Union Army during the American Civil War there were 1 640 000 cases of malaria with 8 100 fatalities.

During the French invasion of Madagascar in 1895, 13 soldiers were killed in action but more than 4 000 died of malaria and during World War I the French and British soldiers were rendered almost inactive by malaria for a period of almost 3 years.

Malaria also attacked those fighting the desert campaign during World War II and actually delayed the Allied invasion of Europe by a considerable period.

Another disease which occurs during the massing of soldiers together, *infective hepatitis,* is an acknowledged problem in army medical history. It was described by Hippocrates 2 000 years ago. It occurred in large numbers during the American Civil War, the Boer War, World War I and World War II. There have been outbreaks in our own army camps in the last decade.

Typhoid fever was another disease that plagued military campaigns, as was dysentery, diseases which spread to the civilian population near military camps.

5.5.2.1 Military nursing

Military nursing service has progressed far from the terrible days at Scutari, and today forms an integral part of military services and defence forces in most countries. It is a sad reflection on our society that wars are not yet absent from the planet earth and that nursing has to be prepared to meet the effects of man's inhumanity to fellow men.

5.5.2.2 International Red Cross

Another tremendous influence on the care of sick and wounded soldiers was that exercised by *Henri Dunant*, who, by chance, stumbled on to the battlefield of Solferino after the battle between the armies of Napoleon III and Austria in 1859. He was so upset by the sufferings of the wounded and dying that he attempted to bring some order into the chaos and to organise nearby villagers to give some form of care to the wounded. This experience was such a nightmare that he wrote an article *Un Souvenir de Solferino* (1862) in which he proposed a plan for dealing with any such future event. This plan involved international cooperation and his writings and efforts led eventually to the foundation, in 1863, of the International Committee of the Red Cross at the Geneva Convention.

This is the greatest humanitarian movement that the world has ever known. Today the Red Cross societies of various nations, united under the International Committee, not only care for those suffering as a result of wars, but provide or coordinate aid for people affected by any disaster. Thus relief is given to those in need as a result of floods, famine, earthquakes and other such occurrences.

5.5.2.3 The nurse's role

The nurse in the military nursing services performs an important role. Her traditional role of providing nursing services to all people, irrespective of race, colour or creed, friend or enemy, is entrenched in the Geneva Convention.

However, the military nursing orders, the military medical and nursing service and the formation of the Red Cross are not entirely responsible for alleviating the lot of the soldier. Advances in preventive medicine, with the resultant immunisation and standards of sanitation, have also played an important part.

5.5.3 Exploration and colonisation

From very early times, men have tended to move away from their place of birth and 'discover' other parts of the world. This tendency was strengthened by the European countries seeking a sea route to the East, 'discovering' Africa and its peoples, 'discovering' the 'New World' (the Americas) and eventually colonising great continents. The 'voyages of discovery' themselves were subject to many health hazards not the least of which was scurvy.

The contact that the early settlers had with the indigenous peoples had definite health implications for both groups. Fighting, for one, brought its own miseries. Furthermore, the settlers came into contact with tropical diseases that were new to them and climates with which they were unfamiliar. Through contact with the settlers the indigenous people, on the other hand, were exposed to infectious diseases that they had not encountered before and many indigenous populations were decimated by diseases such as measles and smallpox, because they had no inbuilt resistance to them.

A positive aspect of colonisation was the more sophisticated health care which the colonising power brought with it. The type of care varied with the stage of development of health care attained by the country that 'exported' its system of health care.

The activities of missionaries often preceded formal colonisation and continued when an area was colonised, contributing greatly to the development of health care systems in the new settlements.

In the process of exporting Western cultural patterns, the colonising powers attempted to educate people native to the colonised land, and with general education went education of health personnel to meet the needs of the times.

6

THE HISTORY OF NURSING IN SOUTH AFRICA*

6.1 Before van Riebeeck

In the early chapters of this book, it was pointed out that explorers found a sea route to India via the Cape of Good Hope. Bartolomeu Dias rounded the Cape in 1488, but did not reach India. However, Vasco da Gama reached 'Calicut' in India in 1498.

It is believed that the Phoeniceans had actually also circumnavigated the Cape in their tiny ships many centuries before. They accomplished this by establishing temporary settlements en route, where their men could rest and procure or produce fresh supplies of food. Centuries later the Portuguese followed a similar policy and established St Helena as a post house on the route to India in 1505.

The first hospital on the African continent was erected in Mozambique, where slaves attended the sick. In 1682 a new hospital, run by the Nursing Brothers of the Order of St John of God, replaced the old one and the standard of care for the sick was greatly improved.

By this time the Dutch too had discovered the sea route to India via the Cape of Good Hope, and eventually established a trading post there.

The loss of life on early trading ships was extremely high and ships were actually lost because the crews were so decimated that there were not enough men left to handle them properly. The journey to the East took about 185 days and the death rate on ships was anything from 30 to 44 per cent. The high death figures were due to overcrowded ships, unhygienic and airless conditions, and lack of sanitary facilities. It is no wonder that typhus was rife. The crews were poorly nourished to start with, the lack of fresh food and water further contributed to illness and to scurvy.

*This chapter is based on the doctoral thesis of Professor Charlotte Searle, which was published as *The history of the development of nursing in South Africa, 1652-1960.*
At her suggestion, and with her permission, a summary suitable for introducing South African nursing history to basic degree and diploma students has been made. South Africa owes such a debt of gratitude to Charlotte Searle for her mammoth research into this subject, as well as for all her contributions to the development of nursing and nursing education in South Africa, that it seems an impertinence to shorten her work in this way. The author, who owes so much to Charlotte Searle, both as one of her students and as a friend, hopes that the taste of what her book offers will encourage nurses to read more widely and to study her book, and that it will spur them on to post-registration study in the subject.
Other sources will be acknowledged in the text, where appropriate, but this introduction serves to acknowledge with gratitude that the bulk of the information contained in it originates from Professor Charlotte Searle.

The Dutch ships, unlike those of the Portuguese, carried barber-surgeons who tended the sick. However, there were too many patients, with the result that they received perfunctory attention. Furthermore, the barber-surgeons had no understanding of disease causation and thus would not have tried to improve conditions aboard ship.

In 1651 the Dutch East India Company decided to establish a refreshment station at the Cape and in 1652 Johan (Jan) van Riebeeck, a surgeon, was appointed Commander of the proposed settlement. He arrived in the Dromedaris on 6 April 1652. Thus the settlement at the Cape and the subsequent development of the South African nation owed its origin to the health needs of a group of people!

6.2 Settlement at the Cape

The beginning of a Cape winter was hardly the most propitious time to start a settlement. The settlers, too, had had a long voyage, were suffering the ills of malnutrition and ill health, and were not strong enough to do much building.

Although one of their priorities was to erect a hospital, the first batch of sick men arrived at the Cape only one month after the arrival of van Riebeeck and his party. Thus the first patients had to be accommodated in tents, which thus formed the first hospital. It was situated on the foreshore, and since there was no equipment, diseases such as dysentery and typhoid fever took a heavy toll. The care given to the sick was poor, there being no staff apart from a superintendent, a young boy apprentice and some convalescent soldiers. Although the great charitable nursing orders were flourishing in Europe and had spread to the American continent, they had not reached the Cape.

Ill officials and women and children of the settlers were cared for at home, since hospitals were regarded as places only for the destitute and homeless during that period of history.

The first White child born in South Africa was the son of the sick comforter, Willem Barentssen Wijlants, on 6 June 1652. Midwifery was a matter for the women of the household, thus the birth of a Hottentot child close to the fort, without the assistance of any attendant, was recorded with surprise on 19 April 1654.

In Holland the practice of midwifery was subject to regulations regarding certification and licensing which were officially in force at the Cape from the time of van Riebeeck's landing. However a sworn midwife was not appointed to the Cape for many years.

The first permanent hospital building was completed in 1656 in the fort, which stood on the site of the present General Post Office. It was thus on the beach.

Diet appears to have played an important part in patient treatment and some degree of sanitary arrangements was attempted. The sick had to supply their own bed linen, and, as there were no bedsteads, had to lie on the floor. Despite all these disadvantages and difficulties, the death rate at the Cape hospital appears to have been low. About 900 patients from the ships were treated each year. Attendants continued to be convalescent patients, who naturally left when they recovered. Some slaves were also used to attend the sick.

Van Riebeeck's hospital served the Company's servants for more than 40 years, although Commander Wagenaar built a new one in 1664, which then also proved too small (34:33).

In 1697 a new hospital was commenced by Simon van der Stel, which was first used in 1699. It was situated almost opposite the present Groote Kerk at the corner of the present Wale and Adderley Streets, next to the Company's gardens. A new feature was that it had bedsteads and was designed for 400 beds, even though it was far too small from the start.

6.3 Overview of the history of South Africa*

What started as a refreshment station and eventually became a nation, obviously underwent many changes as did the rest of the world with exploration, colonisation, the rise and fall in the power of nations, among which there were many struggles and wars. Some colonised countries gained complete independence, others partial independence and some none at all.

Africa, and in particular the southern part which was at the crossroads of routes to the East and West, was no exception. A brief summary of the most important historical events will be given to furnish a background against which to study nursing development.

6.3.1 The Cape

The first arrivals at the Cape found Hottentots and Bushmen inhabiting the area. Exploring parties were sent inland, primarily in search of fresh meat, but 'discovery' of more land was not the reason for these forages. Generally the Company was against colonisation, but the need for more people to grow food made the Company release some of its own servants for this purpose. Thus nine married burghers of Dutch or German origin were settled in the Liesbeeck Valley in 1657. This was really the beginning of permanent settlement at the Cape. Slaves were imported from Madagascar. A Hottentot War occurred between 1658 and 1660, very early in the history of the settlement. The extent of the settled area spread in order to be able to supply more meat and other foods for the visiting ships.

Van Riebeeck sailed east after 10 years, leaving behind an established settlement. Muslims came from India while Hottentots and Blacks became slaves. Mixed marriages took place; thus the Cape Coloureds emerged.

European diseases with which the local inhabitants of this part of Africa had previously had no contact, caused much suffering and death. Because of the threat posed by the French, the Company decided to abandon its opposition to colonisation and Simon van der Stel was sent to the Cape in 1679 as

---

*This section is adapted freely from *A history of Southern Africa* by Eric Walker, and other sources such as the *Reader's Digest illustrated guide to Southern Africa* and *The world of knowledge encyclopaedia*.

Commander to implement the new policy, settling people even further afield and founding Stellenbosch.

The French Huguenots were given refuge in 1688-1689 and were settled among the Dutch settlers, particularly in the Franschhoek area, gradually amalgamating with the Dutch settlers, so that a French Colony never really had a chance to develop. The French brought viticulture to the Cape, while corn, cattle, sheep and general farming was practised.

Gradually more and more expeditions were made into the interior, explorers eventually coming into contact with the Xhosa on the Fish River.

Smallpox appeared in the Cape for the first time in 1713 and killed nearly one quarter of the inhabitants of Cape Town in six weeks. The Hottentots died in hundreds.

Slave trade persisted, as did miscegenation, although manumission, the freeing of slaves, also took place to a limited extent.

The Dutch East India Company came to an end in 1798, and the Cape became the site of refuge for many soldiers, including the French, during the wars that were engulfing the known world.

By 1779 a war with the Xhosa tribesmen had broken out on the eastern frontier. As this time the boers in the area were very remote from Cape Town in thought and way of life. The first British Occupation of the Cape in 1795 was a result of war between half of Europe and the French Republic. As the French were using the Cape, a British attack was not unexpected. This occupation lasted until February 1803.

At the end of the war, the Cape was handed back to the Batavian Republic, which ruled the Cape until 1806, during which time attempts were made to raise the level of civilisation at the Cape.

After the defeat of Napoleon, the British occupied the Cape again in 1806. The colony remained largely based on agriculture. Many social improvements were effected, the first South African lighthouse being built at Green Point. The Royal Observatory was founded in 1824.

Dr Samuel Bailey established a hospital for merchant seamen, slaves and paupers in 1817. This was the first hospital erected for the benefit of the civilians of Cape Town, and not only for the visiting seamen and soldiers. It was erected in the area at present bounded by Prestwick, Alfred, Chiappini and Hospital Streets and named after Lord Charles Somerset. It was taken over by the Burgher Senate in 1821 and moved to Portswood Road (the New Somerset Hospital) in 1852, when the new building was completed (33:34).

Many missionaries from various denominations came to the Cape during this time. The British slave trade was officially abolished by 1823, but slavery was still practised at the Cape until 1833. Border wars continued.

In 1820 approximately 5 000 British settlers landed in the Eastern Cape, thus enlarging the population of the colony considerably. Grahamstown became the centre of the British settler community, while the western frontier moved to the Orange River. English became the official language of the Colony between 1823 and 1828. A new system of justice was also implemented.

The Great Trek began in 1836, and Port Natal was established in 1824. The Supreme Medical Committee, founded in 1803 and later called the Colonial Medical Committee, changed its name to Colonial Medical Council in 1891 (19:445).

Over the years, Cape Town continued to develop as a port and city. It became the seat of Parliament with the formation of the Union of South Africa in 1910. Agriculture continued to flourish and towns such as Paarl, Swellendam, Caledon, George and Mossel Bay were established.

Ports were developed at Port Elizabeth and East London to serve the Eastern Cape and border areas. This area had many problems due to the vagaries of weather, poor soil and of course the border wars with the Black races.

The northern Cape, with Kimberley as its centre, developed sudden prosperity with the discovery of diamonds.

The Karoo, from the Hottentot word meaning 'land of thirst', was originally occupied by almost nomadic White cattle farmers (trekkers, not to be confused with the Voortrekkers of the Great Trek). Many of these farmers were actually the fathers or grandfathers of those who joined the Great Trek. It was predominantly a sheep-farming area with towns such as Beaufort West, Graaff-Reinet, De Aar, Touws River, Laingsburg, Prieska, Sutherland, Victoria West and Oudtshoorn, the land of the ostriches in the Little Karoo.

6.3.2 The Orange Free State

This area was inhabited as a result of an expansion by land-hungry cattle farmers. It became an independent state in 1854, and was involved in a deadly war with the Basuto. Bloemfontein became the main town, and is today the judicial capital of the Republic of South Africa. The Free State became a province of the Union of South Africa in 1910 and of the Republic of South Africa in 1961. It is mainly a stock-farming province, the most important towns being Kroonstad, Harrismith and Parys. Maize (and in some areas wheat) is grown, while diamonds and coal are mined extensively. Development has been remarkable since the discovery and subsequent mining of gold, and towns such as Welkom, Odendaalsrus and Virginia expanded rapidly. Sasolburg is the site of the first oil-from-coal project in South Africa.

6.3.3 Natal

The area was reputedly named by Vasco da Gama, although some doubts exist as to whether he really discovered what is now known as Natal, and not in fact Pondoland. A few ships landed for wood and water in early times. In 1823 Lt Farewell landed there and by 1835 a British Colony was founded. In 1837 Boer Voortrekkers entered Natal and tried to establish a Boer Republic, but in 1843 Natal was formally declared a British Colony, and became separated from the old colony of the Cape in 1856. Natal merged with the other provinces to form the Union of South Africa on 31 May 1910. The leading crops are sugar, maize and wattle bark. Coal is also mined extensively while fisheries is an extensive industry. Natal's history is characterised by many wars with the Zulus, and battles such as Rorke's Drift, Isandhlwana, Gingindlovu are among the best remembered.

Tourism is a flourishing trade along the coast and in the mountains, with the large port of Durban serving the import-export industry. Pietermaritzburg, originally named by the Voortrekkers after Piet Retief and Gerrit Maritz, is the seat of provincial administration. The Church of the Vow, built by the Voortrekkers as thanksgiving for the victory against the Zulus at the Battle of Blood River, is in Pietermaritzburg.

6.3.4 Transvaal

This province is a territory of amazing contrasts, from high mountains to vast plains with rich fertile soil and vast underground wealth in minerals. The Transvaal encompasses a multiplicity of ethnic groups who exhibit many cultural differences. The famous game reserve, the Kruger Nati nal Park is found in the province.

The Voortrekkers arrived in the 1830s, eventually creating the South African Republic with the capital first in Potchefstroom and later in Pretoria. In 1886 George Harrison discovered the gold reef of the Witwatersrand, and a massive gold rush began. There was much political upheaval, petty wars with tribes and eventually the Anglo-Boer War.

The Reef has become a great industrial area with many large, important towns, Johannesburg being the centre of commercial life. In 1947 Dr Robert Broom discovered a prehistoric skull in the Sterkfontein caves. Diamonds are mined, and Premier Mine near Pretoria at Cullinan, produced the famous Cullinan diamond. Pretoria is the administrative capital of the Republic of South Africa and the steel industry at Pretoria and Vanderbijlpark is another giant industrial development.

6.3.5 Anglo-Boer War (1899-1902)

This bitter war between the British and the Republics of the Transvaal and the Orange Free State caused much suffering. At first the British suffered many reverses and lost many troops as a result of typhoid fever but eventually occupied Pretoria on 5 June 1900. Peace was finally signed at Vereeniging on 31 May 1902. The health aspects of this war will be discussed later in this chapter in the section on nursing. After the war the Republics of Transvaal and the Orange Free State were annexed to the British Crown.

6.3.6 Events after Union

The British Parliament passed the Act of Union in September 1909, and thus the self-governing Union of South Africa came into being. 6 700 South Africans were killed when the country supported Britain in the First World War of 1914-1918. However, conflict about this support between the Whites of South Africa led to a rebellion against the government. A campaign was fought against German South West Africa, which led to the German surrender in July

1915. South Africa's own national flag was introduced in 1927, even though it had to be flown alongside the Union Jack.

With the outbreak of the Second World War in 1939, there was again open disagreement about South Africa's involvement, but thousands of men and women nevertheless served with distinction outside the borders of the Union. South Africa also served as a training base for British Commonwealth troops, especially for the Air Force. It was after the end of World War II that the training of the Black nurse really got under way (see section 6.4.10).

The Union of South Africa became the Republic of South Africa in 1961 and left the British Commonwealth. It continued to administer South West Africa (Namibia) until this territory gained complete independence in 1990.

6.3.7 Republic of South Africa

There have been a tremendous number of changes in the short time since the establishment of the Republic. The country has become isolated in many ways, but has also developed its industries to a remarkable degree of self-sufficiency.

National states have been developed for the different Black ethnic groups, some of which have attained independence. New constitutional plans have recently been accepted for the Republic and the future will be determined by those who make tomorrow's history.

6.4 Nursing

The development of nursing in this southern tip of Africa will now be examined against the historical background just sketched. In a work of this nature there are bound to be omissions. The author once again acknowledges indebtedness to the work of Professor Charlotte Searle, without whose initial research and doctoral thesis the nurses of this country would not have known their own history. The events described only include those of the territory which originally formed the Republic of South Africa. Neighbouring territories, such as erstwhile Rhodesia, are deliberately omitted although many of the pioneering nursing work, especially that carried out by the missionaries, overflowed into these areas.

6.4.1 Early stages

The numbers of the sick from ships were large and they were suffering from many diseases, including beri-beri, scurvy, cholera, pulmonary tuberculosis, hepatitis and liver abscesses, bubonic plague and measles. Typhus was introduced into the Cape in 1665 and smallpox in about 1713.

All these conditions require concentrated, skilled nursing, based on a sound knowledge of microbiology, which was not available. At times there were 800 patients in the main hospital, and the total complement of staff for the hospital, its annexes and the Slave Lodge, the barracks and the False Bay Hospital was three chief surgeons, nine undersurgeons (apprentices), one apothecary with one apprentice and 26 'hospitaliers' (soldiers appointed on a semi-permanent basis). The surgeons and their staff no doubt did their best, but the load was too heavy. The so-called 'nursing' was in the main entrusted to convalescents and slaves.

In 1687 'binnenmoeders' (matrons) were directed to be appointed and Aletta Kaisers, the first South African midwife on record, was appointed to the hospital to perform general nursing and midwifery duties.

Descriptions of the hospital of the time present a dismal picture of filth, stench and hopelessly inadequate facilities. The only positive aspect seems to have been the good dietary arrangements which existed generally. These unsatisfactory conditions persisted to the end of the Company's rule.

Jannetjie Ackerboom was appointed as the first 'binnenmoeder'. Her duties were defined in writing in 1700 and included the supervision of the slaves, male and female, who worked in the hospital as bedside attendants, and paying of attention to general cleanliness.

A 'siekenvader' (head male nurse) was also appointed. His duties were similarly defined and included seeing that patients behaved themselves, did not urinate in any but authorised places, and also attending to the cleanliness of the hospital. Six domestic slaves were appointed to attend to the laundry and general scrubbing. This seems a pitifully small number.

The standards of care were poor. Bad management contributed to the unsatisfactory state of affairs and yet it is recorded that the conditions were better than those which existed in Europe at the time!

Home nursing, folk medicine and the care of the poor, sick and aged in the community seems to have been quite good, and was carried out by the women to their own families, friendly neighbours and farmers' wives. According to Theal, a historian quoted by Searle, they were 'highly sensible people'. Hospitalisation for the sick was not favoured, an idea which had been transplanted from Europe. When one reads the accounts of the state of hospitals of the day, then the preference for home care is understood quite easily.

The few sworn midwives who were available were paid a fixed monthly salary by the Company. These women usually came from the Netherlands, although from time to time a few local women were examined and permitted to practise as sworn midwives. Wilhelmina van Zyl (1751), Agatha Blom (1763), Catharina Visagie and Antje Koenes (1788) were among this group. They seem to have been drawn from a stable social class, practising their calling with decorum and efficiency.

6.4.2 The first British Occupation (1795-1803)

During this period the administration of the hospitals changed from that of an institution to serve a commercial organisation to one of a military nature. Medical and nursing practice were not, however, greatly affected.

6.4.3 The Batavian Republic (1803-1806)

The Cape was handed back to the Dutch in 1803. Since the Dutch East India Company had been dissolved, the Batavian Government assumed responsibility for the Cape. The hospital became state controlled and officials and attendants 'public servants'. It was primarily a military hospital, although sailors from passing Dutch ships and civilian paupers were also admitted. The hospital appears to have been well equipped. A working manual for the hospital staff was drawn up, which seems to have laid down sound administrative principles, so that the hospital could have been well managed, and the standard of nursing could also have been good, though records do not clearly state this. When the Cape was surrendered to the British, an era of Dutch health care ended.

6.4.4 From 1807 onwards

The medical practitioners at the Cape were drawn from a wide variety of occupations, not all being qualified to practise. In the Company days, most were barber surgeons, although only a very small number were actually qualified as physicians. Some of the Company officials and employees remained at the Cape, including medical men, who practised as private practitioners. Towards the end of the 18th century a group of university-educated medical practitioners settled at the Cape, while some who had settled during the first British Occupation also remained. These men also had a university education. Statutory control of the practice of medicine was introduced through the establishment of the Supreme Medical Committee in April 1807.

The hospital now became an exclusively military one and the sick poor and sick homeless travellers were admitted to gaols. Sick slaves, attended by other slaves, were catered for in the Slave Lodge, where conditions also appear to have been poor. Some females were employed as attendants in the military hospitals.

The first civilian hospital, Bailey's Somerset Hospital, was established in 1818 (see also section 6.3.1). The state of the hospital, especially after it had been taken over by the Burgher Senate in 1821, left a great deal to be desired. Organisation was poor and nursing was unco-ordinated, much of it being done by a servant class.

Leprosy was fairly common, and eventually a permanent specialised hospital called Hemel en Aarde was established near Caledon for these patients. Some lepers were accommodated at the Somerset Hospital until these were removed to Robben Island in 1846. Although at first the care seems to have been fairly good, it deteriorated rapidly and in 1885 was described as 'shocking'.

Once regulations were introduced for the proper administration of the Somerset Hospital, good standards of care developed and it eventually became an acute general hospital.

As the population grew and the need for more and more civilian services became evident, increasing numbers of patients began to be treated as out-patients by nursing attendants. Hospital nursing gradually extended to the Eastern Cape, where the Kaffir Wars as well as the new settlements created the need for this service.

A series of small general hospitals were set up in Port Elizabeth. In 1856 a temporary hospital was opened in a double-storeyed house in Rodney Street, pending the erection of a provincial hospital. A temporary native hospital was erected in King William's Town in 1856, the Albany Hospital in Grahamstown in 1858 and the Frontier Hospital in Queenstown in 1876.

The medical practitioners, many of whom were attached to the army, played an important part in this development.

Dr John Atherstone, a settler doctor, was a prominent practitioner of the time and did much towards the establishment of medical services in the area around Grahamstown, as did other settler doctors. A group of men and women, some of the latter being the wives or widows of soldiers, gained experience in military hospital nursing and were to form a relatively experienced, disciplined group of nurses. Dr Guybon Atherstone, the son of John, became famous not only for his medical work generally, but because he was the first to use ether as an anaesthetic in the Colony in 1847.

As the standard of living improved, experienced nurses were used by private patients at home, which drained the hospitals of staff. The needs created by the new diamond diggings compounded the problem.

In 1874 the Provincial Hospital at Port Elizabeth obtained the services of two trained and qualified nurses from England, the first of such nurses to be imported. The first Anglican Sister arrived in South Africa in the same year (see section 6.4.6).

Mining activities in the Cape led to the establishment of a new type of hospital for the mostly Black labourers in the mines. These were staffed by White male nurses of the army orderly type.

District nursing for the less affluent members of the community following publications by Dr James Barry was also introduced. Matilda Smith of Bethelsdorp, a widow who became a deaconess, started the first voluntary organisation devoted to the management of a home-visiting service and founded the Cape Ladies' Society for the Relief of the Poor, later the Ladies' Benevolent Society for the Relief of the Poor. Use was made of many respectable widows as visiting district nurses. This service was started 50 years before William Rathbone initiated district nursing services in England in 1859. The Victoria Nurses' Institute, which provided private duty nurses, was established in Cape Town in 1897.

The Voortrekkers had to rely on folk nursing care when they left the Cape.

6.4.4.1 Republic of the Orange Free State

In this area 'medical' and nursing care were both at first provided by 'ou tantes'. Gradually medical practitioners arrived and started practice. In 1874 the Anglican Sisterhood of St Michael and All Angels settled in Bloemfontein and started a small hospital, St George's Hospital (see section 6.4.6). In 1894 the government opened the Volkshospitaal. Diamond-mining activities at Jagersfontein and Koffiefontein led to the erection of hospitals. A small one was also built at Harrismith. Except for the Anglican sisters and a trained nurse at the Volkshospitaal, the nursing was done by untrained attendants.

6.4.4.2 Colony of Natal

After the Natal Colony was annexed to the Cape Colony, a wave of settlers, including doctors, came from Great Britain. The Natal Medical Committee was established in 1856. As in other provinces, folk nursing was carried out by 'ou tantes' and 'monthly nurses'. One room in the prison in Pietermaritzburg was set aside for the sick poor.

Grey's Hospital in Pietermaritzburg was opened in 1857, but care was limited. In 1861 the Bayside Hospital was opened in Smith Street in Durban. However, the staff was unskilled and standards of care poor and in 1879 it was replaced by the New Government Hospital which later became Addington Hospital.

Labourers were brought from India to work on the sugar plantations and some form of medical care was provided for them, but since 'trained' nursing staff was non-existent, most of the nursing care was given by Black and Indian attendants.

6.4.4.3 Transvaal (Zuid-Afrikaansche Republiek)

Again most of the medical and all the nursing care was done by the women of the household and 'ou tantes'. Malaria as well as pneumonia and typhoid fever were probably the cause why trained nurses were being sought and brought to the area, as these were serious health problems.

The discovery of gold (and to a lesser extent diamonds) brought a rush of diggers. Many miners became ill with malaria in Pilgrim's Rest and surrounding areas, as well as Lydenburg, which resulted in the establishment of emergency hospitals.

The Transvaal War (1880-1881) meant that help was requested from the Anglican Sisters at Bloemfontein.

With the discovery of gold at De Kaap and Barberton, thousands of diggers were also attracted to that area. A hotel, the Phoenix, was used as a 'hospital' for the miners laid low with typhoid fever and malaria. Care was given by barmaids. A temporary hospital consisting of corrugated iron shacks was established and two nurses arrived from Kimberley from Sister Henrietta's group in 1886. Care improved rapidly and the sister of one of the nurses came to Barberton to be trained. Sister Henrietta similarly sent a matron and two trained nurses to Pretoria, but language presented a problem as the inhabitants of the 'Republiek' spoke little or no English. In 1890 a new hospital, the 'Volkshospitaal', was opened in Potgieter Street in Pretoria.

The discovery of gold on the Witwatersrand led to more health problems and a temporary hospital, staffed by the Sisters of the Holy Family, was opened in 1888. This was later to become the Johannesburg General Hospital. Other hospitals in the province followed. Training of nurses and other aspects in all these areas are discussed in section 6.4.8.

6.4.5 The Roman Catholic sisterhoods

The first women belonging to a religious sisterhood that came to the country were a group of Roman Catholic nuns of the Assumption Order, headed by Sister Marie Gertrude of the Blessed Sacrament (Notre Mère) who landed in Port Elizabeth en route for Grahamstown in December 1849. These sisters had undertaken a special course in teaching and in district nursing with the sisters of St Vincent de Paul in Paris. They arrived in the middle of a frontier war and rendered great service by visiting the sick and tending the wounded.

In 1867 another order of teachers and nurses arrived in Port Elizabeth from Durban and for 25 years they provided district nursing for the sick poor of that town.

In 1877 the Dominican sisters arrived at King William's Town from Bavaria. Also a teaching order, many were forced to become nurses to meet the health needs of the time. Their order spread throughout the country up to Rhodesia, while helping at Mafeking on the way, and eventually establishing hospitals in the newly established colony.

The Sisters of the Holy Family of Bordeaux staffed the General Hospital in Johannesburg. Mother St Adele was at the head of this group and was also instrumental in starting a three-year training course at the Johannesburg Hospital, issuing a hospital certificate on successful completion of the course. Miss Florence Harvey was the first to obtain this certificate, dated 14 November 1896.

The Holy Family Sisters remained at the Johannesburg General Hospital until 1915, after which they withdrew to take up the running of their own hospitals. By this time many secular nurses, largely from Great Britain, were employed at the hospital.

Besides the hospitals which the Roman Catholic sisters established and staffed in the larger towns, these women played an extremely important part in the field of mission nursing.

As mission work spread throughout Southern Africa and mission stations became established, it was inevitable that the sick would come looking for help. Schools were started, which meant the gathering of many children in one place, who could potentially become ill. At first huts were used to house the sick, but eventually hospitals were built and staffed by nursing nuns. Many of these hospitals supplied a health service which would otherwise have been non-existent.

Many of these hospitals also started training nurses, particularly among the Black women population. Later they were to become provincially and then state subsidised and taken over completely with the development of the 'homeland' policy, with the later national and even independent states. From these hospitals too the comprehensive health policy with outlying clinics was implemented. This type of development was naturally not confined to the

Roman Catholic missions only, but they certainly made a large contribution.

Larger Roman Catholic mission hospitals which also became training schools included Glen Grey in the Glen Grey district near Queenstown, Umlamli at Sterkspruit, St Elizabeth's at Lusikisiki, St Mary's at Mariannhill, St Konrad's at Taung, the Benedictine Mission Hospital and Nongoma and St Patrick's at Bizana.

6.4.6 The Anglican sisterhoods

The first Anglican Women's Order was formed in England in 1845 and a Nursing Order in 1848 at St John's House. This order was the first to introduce hospital training of nurses and also for religious sisters in England, introducing a two-year course at several London hospitals. The pupils paid for their training and midwifery training was also introduced. The All Saints Sisterhood took over St John's House in 1861 and later sent nurses to work in the Somerset Hospital in Cape Town.

Several other Anglican orders came into being about this time. Sister Emma and five associates of the Order of St Thomas the Martyr came to South Africa in 1874 and established the famous Order of St Michael and All Angels in Bloemfontein. One of these five associates, not yet a professed nun, was Henrietta Stockdale, born in 1847 to an upper middle class family. Her father was a minister in the Anglican Church in a small village in England, where she worked in the parish and also helped to raise funds for the Orange River Colony (39:22). She decided to become a mission worker and went to study nursing at Clewer House at Great Ormond Street Children's Hospital. Although she did not undertake a full course of nurse training, she was assigned to teaching on arrival in Bloemfontein. She served her novitiate in Bloemfontein and became a nun of the order.

Sister Henrietta was an exceptional woman who became the Lady Superintendent at Kimberley Hospital and after her retirement from this post conducted the first privately owned district midwifery service in South Africa, in addition to the first agency providing trained nurses to Southern Africa. Encouraged by the church and her order, she travelled extensively in South Africa and back and forth to England.

Both she and Mary Hirst Watkins were members of the International Council of Women, attending the congress in 1899 where a nursing section wat set up. After this, Sisters Henrietta and Mary Hirst Watkins attended a congress of the Matrons' Council of Great Britain and Ireland, where the idea of an *International Council of Nurses* was born. Henrietta Stockdale and Mary Hirst Watkins were the only *registered* nurses at that conference, for no other country had yet obtained state registration for nurses, which Sister Henrietta had achieved in 1891 in South Africa (see section 6.4.18).

The diamond diggings at Kimberley brought many bad health problems, including typhus and typhoid fever. A primitive tent and wattle and daub hospital was erected but conditions were appalling. A wood and iron hospital, the Diggers Central Hospital, was built in 1872. Eventually a provincial

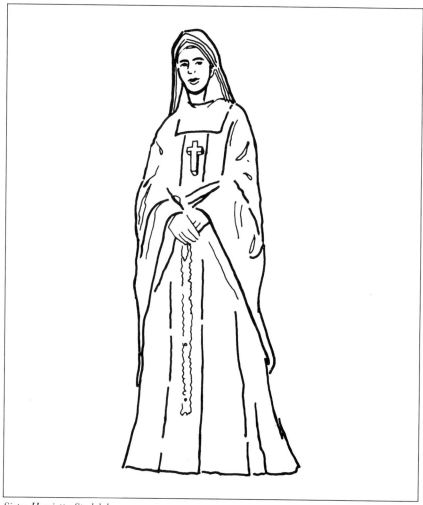

Sister Henrietta Stockdale

hospital was erected next to the Diggers Central Hospital and was named the Carnarvon Hospital. Bishop Webb was asked to find nurses for this new hospital and it was thus that Sister Henrietta and the Sisters of St Michael and All Angels came to Kimberley.

Sister Louise was assigned to the hospital, while Sister Henrietta became a lady visitor, working among the sick poor. She contracted typhoid fever and recuperated in England. In January 1877 she was assigned to assist Sister Louise at the Carnarvon Hospital and was instrumental in starting a training course for the nursing staff who were working with the sisters.

Sister Henrietta was way ahead of the times in her thinking on nursing education, believing that nurses should be trained by the same educational system as that used for teachers, as part of the general education system of the country! Her trained nurses started training others, notably at Barberton in

1887, and Pretoria and Queenstown in 1890.

Sister Henrietta also assisted Sister Mary Agatha to start the training of nurses at the Somerset Hospital. In 1886 Alice Eveline de Beer became the first Afrikaner woman to come forward for training under Sister Henrietta's guidance.

In time the religious sisters withdrew from the hospital at Kimberley, leaving behind a large hospital staff with a training school famous throughout the country, and including a midwifery training section where Mary Hirst Watkins became the founder of modern midwifery training in South Africa, having herself trained at Kimberley.

The sisters of the Community of St Michael and All Angels also provided a district nursing and midwifery service to both the rich and the poor of Bloemfontein and further afield.

Other Anglican orders who nursed in South Africa in the early days include the St George's Sisters (the Grey Sisters) in Cape Town, who were followed and absorbed by the All Saints Sisters. Sister Helen Bowden of this order was instrumental in turning the Somerset Hospital into a well-run hospital. She was followed by Sister Catherine and then by Sister Mary Agatha, who did such yeoman work with the training of nurses. The sisters eventually withdrew from the Somerset Hospital at the end of January 1902.

Again the effect of Anglican mission work in the establishment of hospitals and nurse training schools in remote areas must be acknowledged. Among them are the Jane Furse Memorial Hospital in Sekukuniland, Holy Cross Mission Hospital at Flagstaff, Charles Johnson Memorial Hospital at Nqutu, All Saints Mission Hospital at Encobo, Transkei and St Lucy's Mission Hospital at Tsolo. It is difficult to estimate what a profound part the Anglican sisterhoods and the lay mission hospital services played in the health services of the country and especially in the field of nurse training.

6.4.7 Other missions

The work of various other mission hospitals cannot be forgotten in terms of the establishment of health services and the training of nurses and midwives. All played a significant part. Nearly all hospitals and services provided by various missions became established in answer to local health needs, which became obvious when the Christian message was taken to remote areas.

It is impossible to list them all or even acknowledge the various missionary groups responsible. There are many denominations which were very active in this field. Some of the larger ones which were especially involved in the training of nurses of different categories will be mentioned. In doing so apologies are offered to those that are inadvertently omitted.

☐ *Swiss Presbyterian Group*
  Elim Mission Hospital, Northern Transvaal
  Masana Hospital, Bushbuckridge

☐ *Church of Scotland Mission*
  Donald Fraser Hospital, near Sibasa, Transvaal

Church of Scotland Hospital, Tugela Ferry

☐ *Lutheran Mission Group*
Ceza Mission Hospital, near Mahlabatini, Zululand

☐ *Dutch Reformed Missions*
George Stegmann Hospital, near Rustenburg
Groothoek Hospital, Koringpunt, Northern Transvaal
Philadelphia Mission Hospital, Dennilton
Rietvlei Mission Hospital, Harding
Tshilindini Mission Hospital, near Louis Trichardt
HC Boshoff Mission Hospital, Driekop, Eastern Transvaal

☐ *Others*
Jubilee Mission Hospital, Hammanskraal
Moroka Mission Hospital, Thaba 'Nchu
Shongwe Mission Hospital, Hectorspruit

From this list it is clear that the mission hospitals spread throughout the length and breadth of the land. The age-old link between religion and medical and nursing practice thus still exists today.

6.4.8 State registration

After the Anglican sisterhoods established the first nursing schools, the training of nurses spread rapidly. A completely new type of nurse emerged, namely, one who was trained and aware of her responsibilities to the community. However, each school issued its own certificate and there was no control of practice, a lack which greatly troubled the women concerned.

In England, Mrs Bedford Fenwick launched a campaign for state registration. However, she met with a great deal of opposition especially from Florence Nightingale, who was an extremely influential figure. As a result, England only implemented state registration of nurses in 1919.

In South Africa nurses were to have more success with this movement. Sister Henrietta, a personal friend of Mrs Bedford Fenwick, obtained the support of the medical profession and aided by Dr Callender and Dr Hirst Watkins in Kimberley, pressed ahead and travelled widely to propagate her idea.

It thus came about that the *Medical and Pharmacy Act,* 1891 (Act 34 of 1891) made provision for the licensing and registration of medical practitioners, apothecaries, dentists, chemists and druggists, as well as *midwives* and *nurses.* A Colonial Medical Council was set up and regulations for the examination, certification and registration of nurses and midwives was drawn up. Thus South Africa became the first country in the world to recognise and register nurses by means of the powers granted by Act of Parliament.

This had a tremendous influence on the development of the nursing profession in South Africa. As the other colonies at the tip of Africa gained self-government, they too promulgated regulations for the registration of nurses. At first registration was voluntary, only becoming compulsory in 1944, and even then only for those eligible for registration. It was still possible for nursing to be practised by unregistered persons, there also being no such thing as enrolment of any category.

6.4.9 Nursing during the Anglo-Boer War, 1899-1902

This was a dreadful period in the health history of the southern tip of Africa. Thousands of British troops in military hospitals, and thousands of Republican women and children in concentration camps (established as part of the 'scorched earth' policy of the British) died of typhoid fever, dysentery, measles and its complications and pneumonia. It must be remembered that the same conditions prevailed in military hospitals as those with which Florence Nightingale had to contend in the Crimea, namely lack of hygiene, sanitation and insufficiently trained nurses. There appears to have been general mismanagement of medical services and gross underestimation of needs. It must also be remembered by nurses of the late 20th century that no such things as *antibiotics* and other medications capable of helping to combat diseases of this sort and infections generally, existed.

Prejudicial attitudes existed against using women for military nursing and although 800 trained nurses of the Army Nursing Service Reserve were sent out, this number was hopelessly inadequate. A severe shortage of medical officers and medical supplies also prevailed, while army medical equipment was obsolete. In addition to the dreaded diseases, there were also the wounded to be attended. Locally trained nurses were recruited and gave outstanding service, but the death toll was very high, and many nurses and orderlies contracted typhoid fever.

Unfortunately for the British Army there was no wealthy, powerful woman of the calibre of Florence Nightingale in the Army Nursing Service, and the woman who might have filled this need, Henrietta Stockdale, was a religious sister too old for Military Nursing Service and ineligible for membership of the British Army Nursing Service. What a chance lost, and what a tragedy for the thousands who might have been spared if someone had been able to introduce reasonable hygiene to the hospitals and camps, and if enough good nursing had been available.

'Het Transvaalsche Roode Kruis', the local Red Cross movement, was established in the Zuid-Afrikaansche Republiek in 1896 and members of this movement performed most useful services until the British captured Pretoria. The services of trained nurses were in limited supply and male orderlies did most of the actual nursing. Overseas Red Cross ambulance units were eventually sent out to assist. Emergency hospitals were established, but the services given there were not very satisfactory.

The concentration camps to which thousands of women and children were sent in 1901 were neither large enough nor in any way adequately equipped to cope with the large numbers. The particularly cold highveld winter contributed to the health problems and high disease and death rate, together with poor accommodation, lack of proper sanitation, inadequate bedding, insufficient clothing and food, and a lack of essential supplies and fuel.

There was a shortage of medical personnel, that is, doctors as well as nurses. The ratio was one doctor to 2 238 inmates and one trained nurse to 1 756 inmates! Hospital accommodation was also quite inadequate. Additionally, the misery experienced by the inmates and the fear of being cared for by the enemy compounded a disastrous situation. Eventually the high sickness and mortality rate led to a belated increase in medical and nursing staff. It was during this time that Emily Hobhouse, an English woman and a great humanitarian, did a great deal to bring the dreadful state of the camps and the sufferings and deaths of those confined in them to the attention of the authorities. She was much respected by the female inmates of the camps and did what she could to alleviate their sufferings.

This was a truly miserable period in the health, medical and nursing history of South Africa, with the deaths of 5 853 adults and 22 074 children recorded.

As was the case in the Crimea, the lack of safe environmental hygiene, isolation of infected persons and a supply of the essentials for survival, food, clothing and suitable shelter, were the main cause of this disaster. Furthermore, knowledge of disease causation and its prevention was lacking. The pitifully few medical officers and nurses appear, with few exceptions, to have rendered devoted service to the inmates and the sick in the concentration camps.

6.4.10 Development of nursing among the Black races

Missionaries came from England to the Cape Colony to work among the Hottentots and the Black tribes, and established isolated settlements in the interior. Many realised that there was a need for the care of the sick and many mission hospitals originated from these small beginnings. In 1820 the Rev John Brownlee established a mission station at Chumie, near the present-day King William's Town. He paved the way for all the effective mission work in the Eastern Cape. Educational centres developed as a natural outcome of his work and provided the nucleus of education for Black men and women, which made the eventual education of the Black nurse possible.

In 1856 the first hospital for Black people was established on South African soil. Dr JP Fitzgerald was appointed Superintendent of Hospitals in British Kaffraria. He started his work in King William's Town by opening a clinic for the Black population. The first Black people who were employed by the hospital as interpreters and hospital attendants were men. Dr Fitzgerald wanted assistants who could at least read, write and speak English. The male dominance in tribal life had naturally led to the Black male receiving what education was available. At that time women had little chance of being educated.

In 1857 came the great cattle killing and it is estimated that as a direct result 50 000 Blacks died of starvation in the Ciskei alone. Although the governor had stored food for this event and Brownlee had also laid down large stocks of food, many of those affected by this disaster were too weak to reach the storage areas and died on the way. Relief houses were organised by Dr Fitzgerald and Dr Wilmans, and a relief nursing service was provided by the ladies of King William's Town. Four Black women, the first to be employed as paid hospital nurses, were sent to assist at the hospital and the numbers soon increased.

Dr Fitzgerald obtained the services of Mrs Ellen Parsons, a widow with experience in nursing, with the express purpose of training Black women as nurses. She was appointed in 1869 and carried out her task for 22 years. The training was of necessity rudimentary, reading and writing being included in the 'curriculum'.

Due to their lack of basic education, Black women could not be trained as nurses according to the 'Nightingale pattern' which had been established among women in other parts of the country. Lovedale Hospital prepared the first Black auxiliary nurses with hospital certificates, and the first Black professional nurse, Cecilia Makiwane, was registered in 1908. Dr Fitzgerald and Mrs Parsons must get the real credit for the pioneering work they did in the field of nursing training for Black women.

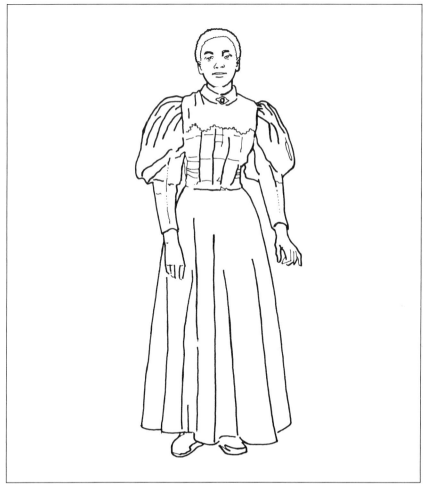

Cecilia Makiwane

Cecilia Makiwane was selected to undertake training at the Victoria Hospital, Lovedale Mission. Her father, the Rev Elijah Makiwane was a minister at the

MacFarlane Mission near Alice, where Cecilia was born in 1880. His views were far-sighted and he had a particular interest in education for all, including women, so it was not surprising that his daughter, contrary to the general ideology at the time, that educating women was superfluous, was given a good general education.

At a time when there was prejudice against Black women entering nursing and when Black people themselves did not approve of unmarried Black women undertaking duties which a nurse had to do perforce, it must have taken considerable courage for Cecilia Makiwane to undertake nurse training. Under Mary Balmer, supported by Dr MacVicar and advised and supervised by Sister Henrietta, the two student nurses had to undergo a strict, rigorous and disciplined training course. Cecilia Makiwane's co-student Mina Coleni completed the same course, but did not register, while Cecilia Makiwane wrote the examination of the Cape Colony Medical Council, and having passed this, became the first Black nurse to be registered in Africa. A statue to her memory was unveiled in the grounds of Lovedale Mission's Lovedale Hospital on 7 May 1977 (39:40,41).

This first registered Black nurse opened up the field of professional nursing to others and at the end of 1988 there were 30 716 Black registered nurses in the Republic of South Africa, according to the statistics of the South African Nursing Council.

Training for Black professional nurses also commenced at McCord Zulu Hospital in Durban in 1924 when the first women with a fair educational background became available, but the training of Black professional nurses in large numbers, sufficient to make a meaningful contribution to the nursing needs of their own people, did not really gain impetus until after the Second World War.

The training of an auxiliary category of Black nurses was also carried out by various organisations and was taken over by the provincial administrations, eventually becoming the enrolled nurse category under the wing of the South African Nursing Council. Nursing assistant training followed.

The first Black assistant matron was appointed in 1958. Basic degree training for Black nurses has been a recent development, being offered at Medunsa, and from 1984 at the University of Fort Hare in association with the Cecilia Makiwane Hospital in the Ciskei. Many Black nurses have taken post-registration degrees in nursing through the University of South Africa. Today many Black nurses hold senior positions in hospitals and health services, and many have specialised in some field of nursing. There are also Black registered nurses with master's degrees in nursing, some of them having done research pertinent to the cultural background of specific health areas, problems and development. Black nurses are employed as lecturers at some universities. Black nurses now also have doctorates and two hold professorial appointments.

The growing contribution of Black nurses to the history of nursing in South Africa is indisputable. Black nurses serve on the South African Nursing

Council and on the Regional and Central Boards of the South African Nursing Association.

It must be emphasised that Black nurses, indeed nurses of all groups, were and still are, subject to the same training regulations, controlled examinations and registration or enrolment. In South African nursing there is no discrimination on the grounds of colour, race, religion or sex.

6.4.11 Development of nursing among the Coloureds and Indians

6.4.11.1 The Coloureds

The Coloured community, a small population group, had its origins in the Western Cape, but other fairly large communities are also to be found in the Port Elizabeth, East London and Johannesburg areas.

Coloured schooling has generally been of a high standard from the beginning, with students gaining access to universities. Nurses are trained at the University of the Western Cape at basic degree level and post-basic diploma and degree level. Many also study through the University of South Africa. Nurses are also trained at diploma level through nursing colleges and affiliated hospitals. The first Coloured woman to be registered as a midwife was Georgina Ada Delicia Judson, registered on 8 January 1918, and the first general nurse, Ella Ruth Gow (later Gow-Kleinsmit), was admitted to the register of the Colonial Medical Council on 6 January 1920. She was also the first Coloured woman to be registered as a general nurse and midwife.

Coloured nurses have also obtained registration in the specialised fields of nursing and many hold senior positions in the various hospitals and health services. At least one has already obtained a master's degree in nursing. They also serve on the South African Nursing Council and the Regional and Central Boards of the South African Nursing Association.

Prof L Evertse (née Muller) was the first Coloured nurse to obtain a doctorate in nursing (D Cur UPE) and also the first to be appointed to a professorial post.

6.4.11.2 The Indians

This is the smallest population group of all. Although Indian women have been very slow to come forward for nursing training, this state of affairs is now improving. Leaders are beginning to emerge and there is no doubt that they, too, will in time make a significant contribution to the history of nursing in South Africa.

6.4.12 Midwifery

The history of midwifery in South Africa has various aspects. The indigenous population was served by the traditional birth attendant and some of their practices were primitive in the extreme, if not positively dangerous. Others, however, were amazingly effective, with an empirical base of generations of gathered knowledge. The treatment of the cord, placenta, puerperium and lactation varied according to the place and the tribe. Maternal and child mortality occurred, but it must be remembered that these also occurred with alarming frequency among the so-called more 'civilised' Western nations.

With the advent of White settlement at the Cape in 1652, birth practices that were observed began to be recorded. The Hottentot woman who gave birth unattended close to the fort on the banks of the river (April 1654) caused so much surprise that it can safely be assumed that Dutch women were used to receiving help and care from others when delivering their babies and during the lying-in period.

It is recorded history that it was the policy of the Dutch East India Company to appoint official midwives to the trading stations in the East and they actually had specific regulations for the purpose of controlling such midwives. These regulations were, in fact, in force as soon as Jan van Riebeeck landed at the Cape. Embodied in them were the requirements that midwives should be in possession of certificates which were granted by examination. In this examination physicians should participate because they had a superior knowledge of midwifery matters (27(a):29). Midwives, then, as now, had to be licensed to practice.

Midwifery services were regarded as a fundamental component of health care. Provision was made for competent assistance during childbirth for those who could not afford to pay. This was free of charge. The regulations were there, but a certificated licensed midwife was not appointed at the Cape for many years, and the women had to help one another to the best of their ability. In the beginning midwifery practice was a service rendered in the homes of the settlers and in the slave lodge in Cape Town. It was in effect either a type of 'private practitioner' or a State District service. The policy of the Dutch East India Company had been to provide sworn midwives who usually came from the Netherlands to practise at the Cape. Some local women were also licensed from time to time.

The administration and organisation of the Cape was considerably disorganised by the First British Occupation from 1795 to 1803. The Batavian Republic authorities, when control of the Cape was once more in Dutch hands (1803-1806), realised that there was a serious shortage of sworn midwives, and planned to establish a midwifery training school there. However, there was again a change of control, the British re-occupying the Cape in 1807. This time the British began to pay attention to the health services, and they set up a Supreme Medical Committee charged with the examination of the qualifications and licensing of doctors and apothecaries. This was later extended to include midwives.

In 1808 the Burgher Senate stated that there were no licensed midwives practising in the Cape, so that any who did present themselves for examination could not have been considered of sufficiently high standard for licensure. Jean Martin, a male ex-surgeon, was refused license by the British authorities to practise as a surgeon, but he was licensed to practise as an 'accoucheur' only.

6.4.12.1 Training – early efforts

The training of midwives on a systematic basis in the Cape actually owes its origins to Dr Johann Heinrich Frederich Carel Leopold Wehr, a surgeon of the Batavian authorities who became licensed to practise as a physician, surgeon and an accoucheur in 1805. He was extremely interested in midwifery and became anxious about the type of midwifery practised at that time by unlicensed persons. According to him unlicensed midwifery was not only inadequate but actually dangerous. In 1808 he wrote a petition to the British Governor-General and Commander-in-Chief of the Cape, Lord Caledon, in which he expressed his gratitude for permission to carry on his medical practice and pointed out that there was a great lack of 'proper and able midwives' in the Colony, he also stated the consequence to the health of mothers and children which resulted from this. He asked for appointment as colonial accoucheur and with it permission to instruct 'an adequate number of midwives for the town of each district'.

This office would also enable him to assist, without charge, the wives and slaves of poor inhabitants. This permission was granted after consultation with the Supreme Medical Committee on 1 August 1808.

The Supreme Medical Committee, in consultation with Dr Wehr, drew up regulations for the training of midwives and the establishment of a midwifery training school. These regulations embodied the following.

☐ The place of instruction, called the School of Theory. This was actually Dr Wehr's house in Castle Street, Cape Town.

☐ The number of women to be instructed at a time being limited to six (four White and two Malay).

☐ A course of lectures to be run over three days a week for a period of three months – three such courses were to be held each year with a gap of a month in between. The intending midwife had to attend three such courses of lectures and practicals and would only be issued with certificates of competency, if deemed fit by Dr Wehr, after which they had to be licensed at the fiscal's office where they had to swear 'a solemn Oath to fulfil the Duties imposed to the best of their ability' (27(a):94).

☐ The slave lodge being named as the practical school.

☐ The School of Theory being open at all times for the future attendance of all who were already licensed to practise.

☐ Midwives had to practise within the strict ethical code which had been drawn up. If found guilty of gross misconduct, lack of attention to their patients or abuse of their positions as midwives, their certificates could be withdrawn and they were forbidden to practise.

Dr Wehr was appointed colonial instructor of midwifery on 1 November 1810 and preparations were made to commence shortly afterwards with such training.

If one examines the above in the light of later developments a few most interesting facts emerge.

- The training pattern was a type of 'study-day-block' system with interspersed practice and was instituted as long ago as 1810.
- The training period occupied three periods of three months each, with one month in-between which made it a minimum of eleven months.
- Provision was made for the updating of practising midwives and the need for continuing education was recognised by the fact that the school was to be open at all times for everyone who had already been certified as competent for practice.
- The school was an educational institution with an attached practical school.
- Students were not paid for their services, but had to maintain themselves throughout the course – tuition was however free.
- The concept of control of ethical standards was recognised.
- Certification of competency was by examinations.

This first midwifery school in South Africa was established on a formal basis 51 years before the St Johns Hospital midwifery school at Kings College in 1861 (27(a):95). The first midwives to complete a full-time course of training did so by 2 August 1813. These women were the first to qualify as professional people in any field of nursing in South Africa and the school was also the first professional school of any kind in South Africa.

Students were taken from country districts as well as from Cape Town. Other groups were trained together with Whites at the school in order to be of service to their own people. Obviously such a small number of trainees could not supply all the needs for midwifery services and many unlicensed persons were practising midwifery. Many women in a sparsely populated rural community had to rely on the services of relatives and friends for assistance in childbirth.

Hospital beds for midwifery

The first hospitals had no beds for midwifery cases. The first official mention of such beds being made available seems to have been at the Albany Hospital in Grahamstown in 1858 (27(a):102). It gradually became standard practice to provide beds in general hospitals for midwifery of an emergency nature.

The next phase – state registration

Sister Henrietta Stockdale, the pioneer of nursing registration in this country, and incidentally in the world, was instrumental in obtaining registration for midwives at the same time as this was obtained for nurses. The passing of the *Medical and Pharmacy Act*, 1891 (Act 34 of 1891) by the Parliament of the Cape Colony made provision *inter alia* for the registration of midwives. Registration was not compulsory. The Act laid down provisions for

- granting certificates of competency in midwifery to those who were holders of certificates or diplomas in midwifery or who subsequently passed examinations by examiners appointed by the Council
- prescribing regulations for training

□ keeping registers

□ disciplinary control.

Regulations for training were promulgated on 31 May 1892. The first persons to register as midwives did so on the grounds of overseas qualifications. The regulations made provision for training under the direction of a medical practitioner. As there were few midwifery beds in hospitals, practical training could be undertaken on district patients or on hospital patients. This made the formal reintroduction of midwifery training possible.

Mary Hirst Watkins is generally recognised as the founder of modern midwifery training in South Africa. In 1892 she was one of the first registered nurses in the world, having trained at the Kimberley Hospital. She continued to work at this hospital and in 1892 was assigned to midwifery district work by Sister Henrietta. The latter had undertaken a course in midwifery training but had never registered as a midwife. Mary Hirst Watkins was trained in midwifery by local doctors and under the supervision of Sister Henrietta and Sister Catherine Booth. The latter was trained in London as a general nurse and midwife and registered in South Africa on 6 September 1892.

Mary Hirst Watkins passed the midwifery examination of the Colonial Medical Council (in Port Elizabeth) in 1893 and was admitted to the register. She was then asked by Sister Henrietta to undertake the training of midwives at Kimberley. This she did, establishing a school which became famous. Her students did so well in the Colonial Medical Council examinations that she was commended on the very high standard of the training which she provided, 16 having been trained by her at Kimberley by the end of 1899. She died in 1905, having been the first nurse-midwifery teacher in South Africa.

Other midwifery training was also instituted. Dr Jane Waterson started a district midwifery service at the Free Dispensary in Cape Town in 1888 and trained midwives herself, but none sat the examination of the Colonial Medical Council and therefore were not registered. Registration of midwives first occurred in the Transvaal in 1896 and in Natal in 1899.

6.4.12.2 The twentieth century

A good foundation had been laid for midwifery training, but much remained to be done. Childbirth was a normal part of everyday life and midwifery care was needed. The sparse population was distributed over wide areas. There were insufficient medical men to meet the obstetrical needs of the community. More and more trained midwives were, and still are, needed today.

The Cape Medical Council was active in its support of midwifery training and the other three medical councils took their cue from them and followed the same policy. Practical training was, at first, undertaken on district, but as midwifery beds became more prevalent in hospitals, training was done both on district and in hospital. This became an established pattern, although the emphasis has shifted largely to hospital training.

Duration of course

Initially the duration of the training course was not laid down by the medical councils, but hospitals made their own rules, the minimum training period required being three months. The medical councils prescribed the minimum number of deliveries to be undertaken by pupil midwives and the number of lying-in patients they were required to care for.

The introduction of a compulsory six-month period of training for registered nurses and 12 months for unregistered persons was brought into being in 1932 by the South African Medical Council which had already had some control over the training of nurses and midwives since its establishment in 1928 some time after the Union. This remained in force until the establishment of the *South African Nursing Council* in 1945. This body was only able to change regulations in 1949 when the duration of the training period laid down was increased from six to nine months for registered nurses and from 12 to 18 months for untrained persons. This has since been increased again in 1960 to 12 months for registered nurses and two years for untrained persons. The emergence of the category of the enrolled nurse, who is also able to undertake training for registration as a midwife over a two-year period, has increased the number of registered midwives available for service to the community considerably.

Regulations

In 1916 the Colonial Medical Council (Cape) gazetted regulations concerning the practice of midwifery by registered persons, this lead being followed by other councils. Training courses had to be approved and training schools were to be inspected.

Financial aspects of training

Midwifery training was paid for by the students and in 1916 amounted to £30-45 for a three-month course of training. Sometimes this amount included board and lodging. Gradually these premiums were reduced and small training allowances were paid to students. When I commenced my midwifery training in 1946 the premium had just been abolished in Cape provincial schools and we received board and lodging and a small training allowance. Private training schools were still demanding premiums as late as 1952 (27(a):325).

Educational standards

The only educational requirement laid down initially was that pupils should be able to read and write. This was changed by the Colonial Medical Council prescribing Standard VI as the minimum educational standard in 1923. This was raised to Standard VII in 1929, to Standard VIII in 1949 and to Standard X in 1960 with some provision for exceptions where prospective students had other nursing qualifications. While Standard VIII remains the entrance educational qualification for enrolled nursing, Standard X (that is 12 years of schooling) is required for the comprehensive course.

The advent of the male midwife (accoucheur)

The decision of the South African Nursing Council to allow males to undertake midwifery training raised protests, although there was also much commendation for the move. Males delivering babies is nothing new, and the intimate care sometimes required from the midwife can be delegated to others. There will never be so many male midwives in training that this will present a problem. In any case, in these enlightened days, the swabbing of females for days after the delivery by midwives has largely fallen into disuse.

Most mothers, who are no longer confined to bed for any length of time after the birth of the child, attend to their own hygienic needs quite adequately. The training of male midwives is in its infancy in this country although not in others, and like all new things, must be allowed to stand the test of time. The fact remains that there is a need for such people, particularly in outlying areas with difficult terrain where the female may find it difficult or unsafe to travel.

6.4.12.3 Recent developments

The integrated course

Perhaps the most significant development in midwifery training of recent years has been the advent of the integrated course combining general nursing and midwifery. Government Notice R3793, published on 28 November 1969, promulgated regulations which made it possible for training schools to prepare general nurses and midwives in one three-and-a-half-year course. The objective of this change was to avoid repetition of portions of the courses which were common to both and to present subject-matter, where possible, on an integrated basis. This was followed by the comprehensive course.

The comprehensive course

Regulations were promulgated for the comprehensive course on 30 September 1983. This course covers at least four academic years and includes General Nursing Science, Psychiatric Nursing Science, Community Nursing Science and Midwifery. This course has phased out other courses as it states 'no person may, after 1 January 1986, be registered as a student at a nursing school for the first time, unless he registers for the course referred to in these regulations' (Government Notice No R2118).

This is an exciting development in nursing education in South Africa. Nursing schools are now linked with universities and nursing education is thus clearly regarded as part of the tertiary education system of the country. The status of nursing colleges is in no doubt and student status can be understood more readily. This does not mean that student nurses will not participate in patient care, but that their learning needs will be taken into consideration at all times. The change should ultimately produce a better registered nurse capable of contributing to the improvement of nursing, and thus health care at all levels.

Changes in emphasis in certain subject-matter

Modern developments necessitate that the emphasis must be changed on various aspects of nursing. In the fields of family planning and mothercraft which have, for a long time, formed part of midwifery training, this is the case. The care of the infant is as vital as that of the mother. The need for family planning is too much part of modern life with the threats that the population explosion has brought to the health of society in general, and too frequent childbearing to the individual woman in particular, to require further discussion here. What is vital is that these subjects are also included in the education of the general nurse and again duplication can be avoided.

Similarly promotive and preventive health care is equally as important to the general nurse as it is to the midwife, and although the emphasis may be slightly different, the midwife's specialised knowledge can be built on that of the general nurse.

Stitching and episiotomies

It is a fact that midwives have often, in the past, been called on to do episiotomies and to stitch perineums. Surely it is then logical to teach them these techniques in the interest of better care of the patient to which they, as midwives, are committed. The teaching of this in the practical field may present some problems, but not problems that cannot be overcome. Simulation techniques take care of the basic procedure and organisation and planning can surely do the rest.

6.4.13 Psychiatric nursing

The attitude to the mentally ill at the Cape Colony was not coloured by such inhuman practices as existed in Western countries, although poor facilities existed for insane paupers. During the jurisdiction of the Dutch East India Company the mentally ill were not ill-treated and only those who became violent were locked up. The more affluent cared for mentally afflicted relatives themselves, incarcerating them when necessary. Those who were not violent were allowed to wander at will. Dangerous pauper lunatics were locked up in the Slave Lodge, where conditions were far from ideal. They were nevertheless not abused and were visited daily by a barber-surgeon. This system was continued during the Batavian Republic.

After the British Occupation in 1806 conditions deteriorated for a while as the seriously insane were admitted to prisons and housed with criminals. When appointed Inspector of Lepers at the 'Tronk' and the Somerset Hospital in 1824, Dr James Barry attempted to bring about reform. He eventually succeeded in building up a pattern of care of the insane with a small core of reasonably satisfactory attendants. James Barry was actually a woman who practised her profession disguised as a man. The fact that 'he' was a woman was only discovered on 'his' death.

When the Burgher Senate assumed the administration of the Somerset Hospital, it already had accommodation for 'lunatics' which it continued to provide. Thus state responsibility for the mentally ill was established early in the history of South Africa.

The Somerset Hospital became the lunatic asylum for the Cape Colony. Treatment was essentially custodial. It was not until the establishment of an asylum for the mentally ill on Robben Island in 1846, that a proper mental nursing service could develop.

A cottage attached to the Albany Hospital in Grahamstown was established for the reception of mentally disturbed patients, and the nurses responsible for attending to the general patients also assumed responsibility for the care of the mentally ill. Many more facilities, including those for the care of feeble-minded children, where humane care was given were also provided. The registration of nurses in 1891 made it possible to train and register mental nurses, and in 1901 regulations for this purpose were drawn up. However, the education of mental nurses got off to a slow start indeed, but courses were eventually established for mental nurses and nurses for mental defectives.

The promulgation of regulations for the training of *psychiatric* nurses took place in 1954, but it took many years before such a course was actually introduced. Today there are 7 636 psychiatric nurses on the register of the South African Nursing Council.

The introduction of psychiatric nursing on an integrated basis into degree courses has given impetus to the training of psychiatric nurses, and a number of nurses prepared in this way have remained in psychiatric nursing. There are now nurses with a master's degree in psychiatric nursing and at least one nurse with a doctorate in this field.

The *Mental Health Act*, 1973 (Act 18 of 1973) which was promulgated in March 1975 was a significant development in the care of the psychiatrically ill, and replaced legislation which had not been altered since 1916.

Many registered general nurses now hold a qualification in psychiatric nursing, 6 517 holding general nursing, midwifery and psychiatric nursing qualifications and 681 general nursing and psychiatric nursing qualifications. This will be further increased with the introduction of the new four-year integrated course.

6.4.14 Community health

The South African Nursing Council has incorporated various aspects of nurse training into post-registration diplomas which has also led to registration as community nurses, and the incorporation of the discipline of community nursing into university nursing courses has also occurred. The latest recognition of community nursing as a basic course has been the incorporation of this nursing discipline into the four-year integrated course, which will further affect the history of nursing in this country.

When one considers the history of nursing in South Africa, it can be seen that the need for the appointment of persons qualified both as nurses and midwives to serve people in remote villages and rural areas of the Cape Colony as *district nurses* was recognised as early as 1885. Acknowledgement must be made of the work of the four 'Vroueverenigings', namely the 'Suid-Afrikaanse Vrouefede-rasie', the 'Afrikaanse Christelike Vrouevereniging' (ACVV) in the Cape, the 'Natalse Christelike Vrouevereniging' in Natal and the 'Oranje Vrouevereni-ging' in the Orange Free State, while a district nursing service was established in 1912 by the Cape Hospital Board. Other voluntary organisations such as the Child Life Protection Society, the King Edward VII Order of Nurses, the South African Red Cross Society, the South African National Council for the Blind and the National Council for the Care of the Physically Disabled in South Africa also played a tremendous part in the establishment of community health care.

All mission hospitals in the country developed some form of district nursing service in the areas which they served, and in most cases trained the indigenous population of the area as nurses and midwives to render such a service. These nurses were especially well equipped to deal with community health problems and health education, belonging as they did to the commu-nities they served.

It is from these roots that the present comprehensive approach to nurse training has evolved. As the country became more industrialised many firms, following world trends, began to pay more attention to the health of their workers, although the full importance of this aspect of community nursing only received recognition with the publication of the report of the Erasmus Commission in 1976.

Courses have been introduced to enable nurses to gain a certificate in occupational nursing issued by the South African Nursing Council.

School nursing in South Africa was established in 1914 and today the nurse bears the brunt of the school health service.

6.4.15 Establishment of the South African Nursing Association and the South African Nursing Council

After the establishment of the Union of South Africa in 1910, the four provincial medical councils continued to exist until 1928 when they were replaced by the South African Medical Council. Registration of nurses was then placed on a national level and nurses and midwives could elect two nurses to the Medical Council.

Dr John Tremble, a medical practitioner of East London, saw the need for nurses to be brought together in a professional association. To that end he persuaded Mr CJ Smith, owner of the Standard Printing Works in East London, to publish a journal especially for nurses, called *The South African Nursing Record,* in 1913. This was run at a financial loss, but Dr John Tremble (who became editor) used it as a means to reach nurses and persuade them of the need to organise themselves. So successful was he that the South African Trained Nurses' Association came into being at the end of 1914. It was as a result of this professional organisation that spectacular changes in nursing affairs in this country, and thus in its nursing history, were eventually brought about.

Right from the beginning the Association worked towards compulsory registration of trained nurses, the improvement of nursing education, the institution of post-registration nursing education, the introduction of more say for the nurses in the running of hospitals, and for the improvement in conditions of service and better socio-economic conditions for nurses.

Membership of the International Council of Nurses, now that there was a properly formed Nursing Association, became possible.

In 1942 a move was made to organise the nurses of South Africa into a trade union. Wise leaders, including Miss Jane McLarty of Johannesburg, saw the dangers inherent in the movement and prompt action by the Association led to the proposal of a Nursing Bill to govern the nursing profession. Mrs VML Ballinger introduced the Bill as a public bill in 1943, and it was subsequently taken over by the government of the day. The *Nursing Act*, 1944 (Act 45 of 1944) was passed and control of the nursing and midwifery professions passed from the hands of the medical profession to that of the nursing profession.

The South African Trained Nurses' Association now became the South African Nursing Association, a statutory body, and another statutory body, the South African Nursing Council, was formed. The *South African Medical and Dental Council* was given representation on the South African Nursing Council and *vice versa*.

Registration of those eligible for registration became compulsory. With the amendment of the Nursing Act in 1970 (Act 31 of 1970) it also became compulsory for all nurses practising for gain to be either *registered* or *enrolled*. The enrolled category included enrolled nurses with a two-year period of training and certification by the South African Nursing Council following examination by that body, as well as enrolled nursing assistants who have a minimum training period of one year, and who are now examined by the SANC . They receive a certificate from the South African Nursing Council, which of course lays down training regulations for all categories of nurse and for diplomas for post-registration courses.

Compulsory membership of the South African Nursing Association was also enforced for all practising registered nurses with the passing of the Nursing Act in 1944.

The South African Nursing Association continues to look after the interests of the profession and its members, while the South African Nursing Council has control of training, examination, disciplinary matters and ethical behaviour of nurses, thus protecting the interests of the people the nurses serve.

The most recent Nursing Act, Act 50 of 1978, brought about direct representation for all population groups on the South African Nursing Council and left the field wide open for the South African Nursing Association to 'do its own thing', while retaining compulsory membership. This Act gives it a firm base from which to negotiate for conditions of service, salaries and any matters affecting the interests of the profession as a whole.

Section 38(a) of the Nursing Amendment Act of 1981 makes provision, in controlled situations, for the nurse to undertake

☐ the physical examination of any persons

☐ the diagnosing of any physical defect, illness or deficiency of any person

☐ the keeping of prescribed medicines and the supply, administering or prescribing thereof on the prescribed conditions

☐ the promotion of family planning, provided that the services of a medical practitioner or a pharmacist, as the circumstances may require, are not available.

The way for the nurse to perform in a wider sphere has thus been legally opened and the South African Nursing Council is at present drafting regulations under this section of the Act which will serve as a guide for nursing practitioners and others.

The South African Nursing Association has used the freedom it gained by the new Nursing Act (Act 50 of 1978) as amended by Act 71 of 1981, to reorganise itself completely. The changes have been to involve nurses from all the national groups directly in the policy-making and regional boards.

The policy of decentralisation of the South African Nursing Association and the division of the country into regions, each with its own regional officer, offices and a regional board, in addition to a Central Board on which each region is represented, has now been implemented. This means that it is now possible for members of the Association to reach their officers with relative ease, and *vice versa*. It also enables them to organise and meet on a regional basis. In a land such as ours, with its vast distances, this is vital. The ability to communicate and exchange ideas in professional workshops, symposia and meetings is the lifeblood of any profession, and regionalisation should make all this possible.

Another important step taken by the South African Nursing Association has been the establishment of a research section at head office. This was initiated by donations from founder members. This development is still in its infancy and should do much to determine local and general needs. Also, research in many areas of our history and cultural health practices will help our future planners to understand the present health patterns and thus to plan more realistically for the future.

The establishment of the *League of Nursing Associations of Southern Africa* (LONASA), which was instigated by actions of the Board of the South African Nursing Association, has also been a milestone in the development of nursing in Southern Africa.

There is also a flourishing publications department at the head office in Pretoria, and a well-stocked lending library. A newspaper, a professional nursing journal, *Nursing RSA*, and a research publication, *Curationis*, are now published by an independent firm.

History has already been made and in a dynamic profession such as nursing major changes will occur, as new needs arise. The new developments will enable the South African Nursing Association and the South African Nursing Council to keep pace with the changing needs of society via its regulations.

6.4.16 Significant developments in the health services in the Republic of South Africa from 1970

There have been so many changes that only the most significant will be mentioned. The following section discuss a few (23:ch6).

6.4.16.1 The national states

Mission hospitals situated in self-governing territories were nationalised and in the seventies became part of the health services of the various states.

A single-tier, hospital-centred, community-directed system with satellite clinics, which formed a comprehensive health service, was developed. Each state had its own Department of Health and Welfare.

Community involvement became an inseparable part of the health services system and specific structures were developed to enable co-ordination with the health services of South Africa.

6.4.16.2 The Republic of South Africa

The Department of Health, later the Department of National Health and Population Development, developed programme budgeting which provided the impetus for

☐ determination of goals and measurable aims for departmental health services

☐ the building up of a strong epidemiological section

☐ identification of gaps in, and allocation of funds for, the rendering of primary health services, such as school health services for Black, Coloured and Indian children and care of the aged

☐ the extension of the national family planning programme

☐ the building up of a network of psychiatric community services

☐ a scientifically founded programme for the combating of diseases such as tuberculosis, all enabling participation and co-operation with other services in the community

☐ laboratory and dental services on a national basis.

In 1977 the *Health Act,*1977 (Act 63 of 1977) replaced the original Act, which had been drawn up in 1919 after the influenza pandemic which claimed the lives of 150 000 people in the then Union of South Africa. Although the original Act had been amended many times, it was outdated and a new Act was necessary. This new Act has made provision for a National Health Policy Council, and a Health Matters Advisory Committee, with sub-committees. The Act defines the functions of the Department of Health and Welfare, the provincial administrations and the local authorities regarding health matters, and makes it possible for far greater co-operation and co-ordination to be achieved between these bodies.

Nurses are involved in many of the sub-committees established under this Act and its regulations, apart from the specific Sub-committee on Nursing, which with the exception of the chairman is composed entirely of nurses.

A National Health Services Facilities Plan, announced in November 1980 by the Minister of Health, forms a basis for the extension of future health services and facilities. The basic policy of this plan states that there should not only be facilities for rendering health services, but that services should actually be delivered and funds be provided for the development of a comprehensive health service.

6.4.17 Developments in nursing education

According to Charlotte Searle, nursing education may be called a 'production line' for the skilled nurses required by a community, but as this book concentrates on basic developments, only a list of the most important developments will be given.

All the developments have meant that the education of nurses has had to be drastically revised from time to time. The South African Nursing Council has been concentrating on this aspect continually, as is evidenced by the announcement of the new integrated course in 1982. More advanced and specialist courses have been introduced, while some that have outgrown their usefulness have been scrapped.

Nursing education in the Afrikaans medium was introduced in the Orange Free State in 1925, a development which was brought about mainly due to Miss Elizabeth Lotz, the Matron of the Volks National Hospital, Bloemfontein. In 1920 Miss A Schoeman, a sister in that hospital, took over the coaching in Afrikaans in the wards.

In 1929 Miss Corrie Loopuyt pioneered the teaching of nurses through the medium of Afrikaans at the Somerset Hospital, Cape Town. This was followed by Miss Anna Schoemann at the Far East Rand Hospital, Miss Alida Beyers at Pretoria Hospital, Miss W le Roux at Boksburg and Mrs C Searle in Klerksdorp.

The preparation of nurse-educators through the medium of Afrikaans was pioneered by the University of Pretoria.

A 'block system' of education for nurses was introduced into South Africa by Miss E Pike at Groote Schuur Hospital in June 1934.

Colleges of nursing were established by various provincial administrations responsible for nursing education. The first was established towards the end of 1945 and later named the BG Alexander College of Nursing in honour of Bella Gordon Alexander RRC, one-time matron at the Johannesburg General Hospital, who made nursing education her life's work.

On 1 April 1947 the Transvaal Provincial Administration appointed a nurse to the Department of Hospital Services and soon other provinces followed suit. All four, as well as the Department of Health, now have a corps of nurses working at head-office level.

Cape Town University and the University of the Witwatersrand were the first two universities to provide courses for nurses at university level with the introduction of post-registration diplomas in nursing (nurse-educator) courses in 1933.

In 1956 the University of Pretoria introduced the first generic degree course in nursing at a South African university. Since then many other universities have followed suit, and in 1966 Dr C Searle was the first nurse in South Africa to be awarded a doctor's degree (in sociology). As has already been stated, her doctoral thesis formed the basis for most of this chapter on the history of nursing in South Africa.

Many universities have also graduated nurses with honours and masters as well as some doctoral degrees. The first doctorate in nursing was conferred on JM Mellish on 18 September 1976, also by the University of Pretoria.

In 1975 the University of South Africa started to offer nursing degrees. These are, of course, post-registration degrees, which have met the needs of many registered nurses who could not attend residential universities for a variety of reasons.

Perhaps the most exciting development in nursing education is the planned linking of nursing colleges with universities, so that nursing education may take its proper place in the stream of general education, something that certainly would have gladdened the heart of Sister Henrietta Stockdale.

The first professor of nursing, Professor Charlotte Searle, was appointed to the chair of nursing at Pretoria University on 1 March 1967.

The first male nurse, Dr CT Rautenbach, obtained a doctorate in nursing in 1981 at the University of Port Elizabeth.

Nurses in South Africa have entered the fields of writing and research in both official languages and as stated elsewhere, a research unit has been established at the central office of the South African Nursing Association in Pretoria.

6.4.18 A few figures who have contributed to the development of nursing in South Africa*

This section does not pretend to be complete, nor will it give many details of the people mentioned, but it is felt that a brief note on some of the outstanding figures who have helped to shape the history of nursing in South Africa is necessary. Important nursing personalities such as Sister Henrietta Stockdale, who was discussed in some detail in a previous paragraph, will be omitted.

☐ *Mrs HC Horwood* followed Miss BG Alexander as General Secretary of the South African Trained Nurses' Association. She was also the second editor of the *South African Nursing Journal*, retiring from that post on 31 March 1945.

☐ *Mrs Sharley Mary Cribb*, who followed Mrs Horwood as organising secretary of the South African Trained Nurses' Association, bore the brunt of the campaign for the Nursing Act, travelling widely and addressing meetings of nurses throughout the country. She was appointed the first organising

---

*Tributes to many more and more details will be found in the publications of the **SAN Association's** *Nurses of Distinction*.

secretary of the South African Nursing Association. She had vision, drive and an enormous capacity for hard work. Her death in 1946 was a tragic blow to the new Association.

☐ *Miss Constance Ann Nothard*, RRC, was Matron-in-Chief of the South African Military Nursing Service during World War II and was actively engaged in the campaign for a Nursing Act, becoming the first President of South African Nursing Council, an office which she filled with great distinction for several terms of office. She was also very active in Association affairs.

☐ *Miss Bella Gordon Alexander*, RRC, was at one time Matron of the Johannesburg General Hospital, Honorary Organising Secretary of the South African Trained Nurses' Association and later President for several terms of office of that Association. She played a leading role in building up the Association, in extending the range and scope of its activities both nationally and internationally, and in nursing educational development.

☐ *Miss Jane McLarty*. Matron of the Johannesburg Non-European Hospital and later of Baragwanath Hospital, was very active in the movement to block trade unionism, and to have a Nursing Act promulgated. She was active in the field of education of Black nurses and President of the South African Nursing Association from 1944 to 1946.

☐ *Miss M Greta Borcherds*, RRC, a most distinguished nurse who eventually retired from the Johannesburg Hospital as its Chief Matron, also played a part in the efforts to get a Nursing Act, and served two terms as President of the South African Nursing Association, presiding over the Golden Jubilee Celebrations in 1964 with charm and dignity. Miss Borcherds also served on the South African Nursing Council. She was charged with the responsibility of developing the first South African Nursing College.

☐ *Miss JC Child*, a product of the Nightingale School, had the vision and enthusiasm to collaborate wholeheartedly with Dr John Tremble, founder of the South African Trained Nurses' Association, and so provided the much needed nursing leadership to launch the professional association of nurses in South Africa (27(b):17).

☐ *Miss Sybil Marwick*, at one time President of the South African Trained Nurses' Association, retired from nursing as Chief Nursing Officer of the Cape Provincial Administration Hospital Services Department, having also been Chief Matron of Groote Schuur Hospital.

☐ *Miss Iris I Marwick* is another distinguished nurse who made a tremendous contribution to psychiatric nursing and the education of psychiatric nurses in South Africa. She first trained as a general nurse and midwife at Grey's Hospital, Pietermaritzburg. Miss Marwick was a pioneer of the open-door policy for psychiatric patients, starting an occupational therapy department at Fort Napier Hospital, which expanded into the important service it is today in psychiatric hospitals and was eventually part of the establishment of Tara Hospital. She was the first psychiatric trained nurse to qualify as a nurse tutor and was well-known internationally for her contribution to psychiatric nursing.

☐ *Prof Charlotte Searle* (née Pietersen) was born in the same year that Florence Nightingale died. She was trained as a general nurse at Kimberley hospital (Sister Henrietta's hospital) and in midwifery at the Mother's Hospital, Durban, whereafter she graduated with a BA in Social Work from Unisa in 1947. During this time she also completed her Sister Tutor's Diploma (1946) at the University of the Witwatersrand. In 1952 Prof Searle completed her MA (Sociology) at the University of Pretoria, as well as her Diploma in Hospital Administration. Prof Searle then qualified as Health Visitor and School Nurse from Pretoria Technical College in 1960 and went on to obtain her DPhil *cum laude* from Pretoria University in 1965 with the thesis *History of the Development of Nursing in South Africa 1652-1960*, whereby she became the first nurse to earn a doctorate in South Africa. She is an untiring writer and is married with one daughter.

Among her other achievements are the active role she played in the South African Trained Nurses Association, especially in the fight against trade unionism. She is also a founder member of the South African Nursing Council, and was President of the South African Nursing Association from 1973-1983. Furthermore she was and is a member of the South African Nursing Council from its inception in 1945 (with a break of 2 years) until the present time.

Prof Searle has undertaken many study tours overseas.

She pioneered the training of nurses at degree level at South African universities, and promoted the first nurses to obtain higher degrees (masters and doctoral) at the University of Pretoria, and established departments of nursing in many South African universities. Furthermore she also played a key role in the development of training for nurse tutors in Afrikaans.

The Department of Nursing at UNISA was started by Prof Searle, and this made higher education available to nurses throughout the country who were too far removed from the residential universities, or who could not leave their posts and their families.

She was a prime mover in the affiliation of nursing colleges to universities for the education of basic diploma students in nursing.

Prof Searle has received many awards and this short summary cannot do justice to a truly remarkable nurse leader who is, above all, a nurse educator.

☐ *Professor Patricia Hilda (Paddy) Harrison* served the profession faithfully for many years as President of the South African Nursing Association for a term of office and as Vice-President for several terms. She was the first professor of nursing at the University of Cape Town and also served on the South African Nursing Council.

☐ *Dr AS Latsky*, second President of the South African Nursing Council, eventually retired as Chief Nursing Officer of the Transvaal Provincial Administration Department of Hospital Services, receiving a doctorate, Honoris Causa, from the University of Potchefstroom. She also served her profession actively as a member of the Board of the South African Nursing Association.

☐ *Miss Doreen Henrietta Radloff* served as organising secretary and later (1947–1980) as Executive Director of the South African Nursing Association. She is well known to many nurses, and did a tremendous amount to build up the South African Nursing Association from small beginnings into the large organisation of today. She took over only a short time after the passing of the Nursing Act. Her efforts on behalf of members were untiring, and her contribution to professional development immeasurable.

☐ *Miss AW (Nancy) Simpson*, who also retired as Chief Matron of Baragwanath Hospital, made a tremendous contribution to the education of Black nurses and to their professional development. She also served as President of the South African Nursing Association from the end of 1950 until November 1952.

☐ *Miss BL Alford* trained at Victoria Hospital Wynberg, doing midwifery at Peninsula Maternity Hospital and later Health Visiting and School Nursing. She will be best remembered as editor of the *SA Nursing Journal* from 1960 until 1979 when she retired, working in a part-time capacity as editor of the *SANA's*, then professional quarterly publication *Curationis*, and as liaison officer for the Association's monthly newspaper *Nursing News* which succeeded the *SA Nursing Journal* in 1978. Miss Alford was awarded the CJ Smith medal in 1975 for her outstanding contribution to nursing.

☐ *Mrs ME Venter* served two terms of office as President of the South African Nursing Council and retired from nursing as Chief Nursing Officer of the Orange Free State Provincial Administration Hospital Services Department. She was also well known for her role as inspector of training schools for the South African Nursing Council. She served her profession devotedly as a member of the Board of the South African Nursing Association.

Other names that must be mentioned are Cecilia Makiwane, the first Black nurse to be admitted to a State Register for nurses or for midwives, and Mrs Georgina Judson, the first Coloured nurse to pass a final examination conducted by a state registration authority in South Africa and to be admitted to a State Register for nurses or for midwives.

The present President of the South African Nursing Association is Miss Odelia Muller. The present President of the South African Nursing Council is Prof W Kotzé of the University of Port Elizabeth.

Basically, from the beginning of time, the specific health needs of people are being met by other people. This remains fundamental as life from before birth until death continues on the planet earth. New health hazards appear as old ones are conquered, thus nursing history will never be complete, while human beings survive.

The history of nursing both in South Africa and in the wider world continues to undergo change in keeping with the health needs of the times and the areas in which nursing is practised. It is hoped that this basic history will whet the appetites of readers and stimulate them to further study.

Bibliography

Books

1. Baly ME 1973 *Nursing and social change* London: Heinemann.

2. Bowra CM 1966 Classical Greece in *Great ages of man* The Netherlands: Time-Life International.

3. Baartman DTN 1983 *Traditional and modern approaches to the health care of pregnant women in Xhosa society* Unpublished MA (Cur) Unisa dissertation.

4. Casson J 1966 Ancient Egypt in *Great ages of man* The Netherlands: Time-Life International.

5. Charley IH 1954 *The birth of industrial nursing* London: Baillière.

6. Colton J 1966 Twentieth century in *Great ages of man* The Netherlands: Time-Life International.

7. Davidson B 1966 African kingdoms in *Great ages of man* The Netherlands: Time-Life International.

8. Dolan JA 1968 *History of nursing* London: Saunders.

9. Donahue MP 1985 *Nursing, the finest art* St Louis: CV Mosby.

10. Dowley T 1988 (organising ed) *The history of Christianity* Cape Town: Struik Christian Books.

11. Freemantle Anne 1966 Age of faith in *Great ages of man* The Netherlands: Time-Life International.

12. Gay P 1966 The age of enlightenment in *Great ages of man* The Netherlands: Time-Life International.

13. Hadas M 1966 Imperial Rome in *Great ages of man* The Netherlands: Time-Life International.

14. (a) Hale JR 1966 Renaissance in *Great ages of man* The Netherlands: Time-Life International.

    (b) Hale JR 1966 Age of exploration in *Great ages of man* The Netherlands: Time-Life International.

15. Harper HH (quoted by Baartman) 1965 *Review of physiological chemistry* California: Large Medical Publications.

16. Herodotus 1954 *The histories* Harmondsworth: Penguin (translated by Aubrey de Sélincourt).

17. *The Holy Bible* 1979 New International Version Cape Town: Bible Society of South Africa.

18. Kindersley D Ltd 1984 (ed & design) *Quest for the past* Pleasantville New York, Montreal: Readers Digest Ass Inc.

19. Laidler PW & Gelfand M 1971 *South Africa: its medical history* Cape Town: Struik.

20. Leonard JN 1966 Ancient America in *Great ages of man* The Netherlands: Time-Life International.

21. Lissner I 1960 *The living past* London: The Reprint Society (translated from German by arrangement with Jonathan Cape).

22. Margotta R in P Lewis (ed) 1968 *An illustrated history of medicine* Feltham: Paul Hamlyn.

23. Muller O 1982 *Important developments in public health services in the RSA during the seventies* Cape Town: King Edward VI Trust.

24. Piggot S (ed) 1962 *The dawn of civilisation* London: Thames & Hudson.

25. Schafer EH 1966 Ancient China in *Great ages of man* The Netherlands: Time-Life International.

26. Schulberg L 1966 Historic India in *Great ages of man* The Netherlands: Time-Life International.

27. (a) Searle C 1965 *The history of the development of nursing in South Africa* Pretoria: The South African Nursing Association.

    (b) Searle C 1964 *Overview of nursing education in South Africa 1914-1964* Pretoria: South African Nursing Association.

    (c) Searle C 1964 *Testimony to fifty years of service* Pretoria: South African Nursing Association.

28. Shyrock RH 1959 *History of nursing: an interpretation of the social and medical factors involved* Philadelphia: WB Saunders.

29. Walker EH 1968 *A history of South Africa* (rev impr) London: Longmans & Green.

30. Ward K (ed) 1987 *Jesus and His times* Pleasantville, New York, Montreal: Readers Digest Association.

31. Woodham-Smith C 1952 *Florence Nightingale* London: The Reprint Society.

32. *World of knowledge encyclopaedia* 1971 London: Heron Books.

Articles

33. De Villiers JC & Keyser AL 1983 (29 Jun) Lost hospitals of the Cape *South African Medical Journal* (special ed).

34. Ferguson M 1979 (15-29 Nov) Reflections on the teaching practice of nursing *Nursing Times* (occasional paper).

35. Greene RC 1987 (Aug) The epidemics that delayed D Day *Nursing RSA* Vol 2 No 8 Cape Town (Reprinted from *Medical News Tribune* Vol 4 No 4 (1986 13 Nov)).

36. Iveson-Iveson J 1982 (Mar-May) History of nursing *Nursing Mirror*.

37. Karlsson EL & MoPoanto KEM 1986 (Mar). The traditional Healer *Nursing RSA* Vol 1 No 2 Cape Town (Reprinted from *SA Journal of Continuing Medical Education* 2).

38. Searle C Career Woman *Nursing RSA* Vol 2 No 4 Cape Town.

39. Tibbett J 1987 (Jan) Cecilia Makiwane *Nursing RSA* Vol 2 No 1 Cape Town.

40. Van Rensburg HCJ 1981 (Sep) Die aard en stand van tradisionele Westerse of stammedisyne in Suid-Afrika *Curationis* Pretoria: South African Nursing Association.

Dictionaries

41. Chambers 20th Century Dictionary 1983 Edinburgh.

Index